SIR JAMES SPENCE

The origins and evolution of a legacy in
Newcastle upon Tyne. 1923 to1997

HANS STEINER, ELIZABETH GREENACRE and ALAN CRAFT

(signature)

BLACKTHORN PRESS

Blackthorn Press, Blackthorn House
Middleton Rd, Pickering YO18 8AL
United Kingdom

www.blackthornpress.com

ISBN 978 1 906259 46 4

CONTENTS

The Legacy of Sir James Spence

FOREWORD: JOHN WALTON

My abiding recollection of Spence is of a man of extraordinary charisma, and at times electrifying personality.

I first met him when I was a medical student, and like many of my fellow students I worshipped him. There is no doubt that he was one of the key influences in my early career and a continuing inspiration for over seventy years.

He was a fine doctor, a superb teacher, an outstanding role model and a very great man. One of his great insights was to recognise the importance of the mother in the care of a sick child. I remember well his ability to talk to mothers and put them at their ease. Admitting mothers with their sick children is standard practice today across the world, but it was Spence who had the vision to see how important this would be for both the child and the mother.

There is no doubt that Spence was one of the great doctors of the first half of the twentieth century and his influence shaped the way that we care for sick children today. Indeed, when he received his wholly deserved knighthood, *The Lancet* wrote, 'His flow of ideas, always arresting and often strangely right, made him one of the most valued members of our profession.'

It is timely now, some sixty years after his premature death, that we review the impact he has made, and Hans Steiner and his colleagues are to be congratulated on capturing the essence of a great man in this superb publication.

John, Lord Walton of Detchant, Kt TD MA MD DSc FRCP Fmed Sci

Former Professor of Neurology and Dean of Medicine, University of Newcastle upon Tyne

Former Warden, Green College Oxford

Former President, British Medical Association, General Medical Council, Royal Society of Medicine, Association of British Neurologists and World Federation of Neurology

PREFACE

This is a new evaluation of the legacy of Sir James Spence, the first full time Professor of Child Health in England.

He was a pioneer in the development of paediatrics during the 1920s-40s, including the understanding of the family, social and community dimensions of the speciality.

The Babies Hospital was the principal clinical base where he developed and implemented his ideas about the appropriate care of the youngest sick children in our communities. He was the first physician in the country to welcome mothers on a regular basis to come into residence to participate in the care of their children under the supervision of the nurses and he developed systems of care to meet their special needs.

As he came to understand the importance of the family and social/environmental factors that affect the health and determine the origin and outcome of childhood diseases, he initiated studies to elucidate their nature and significance.

The last appraisal of his legacy was published 41 years ago in 1975 by his successor, Professor Donald Court.

The present study includes little known and some entirely new data and insights about his clinical activities, teaching and researches. These are based on a study of the Annual Reports of the West End Day Nursery (1919-1924), where 'J.C." as he was known to everyone, started his work with children in Newcastle, and the Annual Reports of the first Babies Hospital throughout its life (1925-1945).

This information is unique as it is based on J.C.s own accounts, as he was responsible for writing the medical components of the Reports as well as extensive commentaries about new ideas, findings and practices. By quoting many verbatim it has been possible to 'hear' the progression of his thoughts, like a vivid voice from the past.

His legacy continued to shape the development of child health and paediatrics in Newcastle after his death in 1954. Those who followed him in Newcastle embraced the ethos that he initiated and adapted conditions, clinical practices, teaching and research to meet the new priorities that emerged in these specialities.

As infections and malnutrition gave way to more specific organic and chronic conditions, disabilities, developmental and behavioural problems and finally the damaging consequences of child abuse and neglect, new residential hospital facilities for parents and their children were made available to participate in the assessment and care of children with these problems.

An analysis of the Admission Records of the later Babies Hospital at Leazes Terrace which closed in 1976, as well as the Audit and Progress Reports of the specialist Mother and Child and Family Units, that were maintained in other hospitals in Newcastle for another two decades until 1997, bear testimony to the fruits of his legacy.

Sir James Spence played a pivotal role locally, nationally and internationally in the development of a greater understanding of the needs of children and their families.

This study has shown that most of his ideas have stood the test of time. He was very much a physician in tune with the mores of his era, some of which, inevitably, have now been superseded.

He was an early pioneer who inspired significant progress in the understanding and management of childhood diseases in the context of their social/environmental conditions and the pivotal role of the family in their children's welfare.

ACKNOWLEDGEMENTS

We are particularly grateful to Sophie Addley (Steiner) for typing and editing the manuscript, to Nikky Steiner for producing the colour coded graphs, and to Matthew and Emily Steiner for technical help and support. Also, Dr Carole Kaplan, consultant child psychiatrist and Dr Trian Fundudis, consultant child psychologist from the Nuffield Psychology and Psychiatry Unit for Children and Young People for their helpful comments.

The following colleagues from Newcastle upon Tyne, all now retired, have contributed information and recollections about various aspects of the study:

Miss Christine Cardose, nursery nurse, Mother and Child Unit at the Fleming Memorial Hospital for Sick Children and Family Unit at Newcastle General Hospital.

Professor Allan Colver, Community Child Health, University of Newcastle upon Tyne.

Dr Simon Court, consultant paediatrician.

Mrs. Anne Craft, staff nurse and later Chief Nursing Officer at the Royal Victoria Infirmary.

Miss Marge Craig, community development officer, Riverside Child Health Project.

Dr Mike Downham, Senior Lecturer in Child Health, University of Newcastle upon Tyne.

Miss Sue Jackson, social worker, Fleming Memorial Hospital for Sick Children.

Dr Camille Lazaro, senior lecturer in paediatric forensic medicine, University of Newcastle upon Tyne and consultant paedatrician.

Dr Kurt Schapira, consultant psychiatrist.

Mr John Wagget, consultant paediatric surgeon.

We are also grateful to Mrs. Audrey McIntyre, personal assistant to Professor Sir Alan Craft, for recent help with locating references and to Mrs. Julia Temple, medical secretary to the Mother and Child Unit, Fleming Hospital and the Family Unit, Newcastle Hospital, for 20 years (1977-1997), who was responsible for assisting in the extensive communications with health and social services and the production of the numerous audit and paediatric reports for the legal proceedings during those years.

We would like to acknowledge the debt that we owe to the many publications about the people, the events and the analyses that we have included in our manuscript and in particular three publications, from which we have quoted at some length: "The Purpose and Practice of Medicine", which includes a Memoir by Sir John Charles and a Selection of Sir James Spence's writings. Oxford University Press, 1960. Ridley U. "The Babies Hospital. Newcastle upon Tyne". Andrew Reid Company.1956. James and Joyce

Robertson. "Separation and the Very Young". Free Association Books. London.1989.

We are grateful to the Newcastle Health Care Charity for a generous donation towards the costs of publication and distribution. All income from sales will be donated to The Great North Children's Hospital Foundation, Newcastle upon Tyne.

Finally, we would like to acknowledge the unfailing courtesy of Alan Avery of the Blackthorn Press who gave us the essential advice in order to complete the preparation of the manuscript for publication and the efficiency with which this was achieved.

The photographs

The black and white photos from 1926-1945, are taken from the Annual Reports of the Babies Hospital and Lady Ursula Ridley's Memoir of 1956[3].The photos of the Children's Clinic of the Royal Victoria Infirmary in 1946 were taken by that hospital's Photography Department and that of Dr Cooper by the Newcastle University Audiovisual Centre.

The sources of all the photographs are recorded in the manuscript.

ABOUT THE AUTHORS

Dr Hans Steiner, BA (Hons Open), MD, FRCP, DCH, D Obst RCOG, trained in Newcastle upon Tyne, including the Babies Hospital in Leazes Terrace. He then pursued a career as First Assistant to Professor Donald Court (successor to Sir James Spence), Senior Lecturer in Child Health and consultant paediatrician in Newcastle and Northumberland (1974-1994).

Miss Elizabeth Greenacre, SRN, RSCN, trained in Newcastle, including the Babies Hospital in Leazes Terrace and was formerly a staff nurse and sister in charge of the Mother and Child Unit at the Fleming Memorial Hospital for Sick Children and the Family Unit at Newcastle General Hospital. (1977-1997).

Professor Sir Alan Craft, MD, FRCP, FRCPH, FMed Sci, is a graduate of the Medical School of Newcastle upon Tyne (1969) and completed his paediatric training in Tyneside. He was a consultant in the area with a special interest in paediatric oncology and was Sir James Spence Professor of Child Health (1993 - 2007). He is a former President of the Royal College of Paediatrics and Child Health (2003 - 2006).

ILLUSTRATIONS

Figure 12a and b. The Babies Hospital
Outpatient's notes and exchange of letters between Sir James Spence and family doctor 1939

Figure 13. Sources of Referral to the Babies Hospital
1926-1944

Figure 14. The Babies Hospital and Mothercraft Centre
Visitors to the hospital. Dr G. Brewis (Honorary Assistant Physician), a visitor, Lady Ridley and Dr James Spence
Annual Report. 1937

Figure 15. The First Annual Report 1925 - 1926

Figure 16. The finances from the First Annual Report. 1925-1926

Figure 17. The Princess Mary Maternity Hospital. 1948
Baby's cot at the mother's bedside
Photography Department, King's College, Newcastle

Figure 18. The Babies Hospital, West Parade 1937-1939
and Blagdon Hall, Northumberland 1940-1945
The changing pattern of diagnoses

Figure 19. The Babies Hospital at Blagdon Hall, Northumberland 1939 – 1945
Annual Report 1940

Figure 20. The Babies Hospital 1939 - 1945
Nurses and patients in the garden at Blagdon Hall
Lady Ridley's Memoir.1956

Figure 21. The Babies Hospital, Blagdon Hall 1939 – 1945
Nursery for long stay patients
Lady Ridley's Memoir. 1956

Figure 22. The Babies Hospital
Lady Ridley, Dr Spence and Miss Cummings, who was the matron from 1929 to 1942
Lady Ridley's Memoir. 1956

Figures 23a, and b. The Babies Hospital at Leazes Terrace 1966
The terrace houses and the park across the road
Audio visual Centre. Newcastle University

Figure 24. The Babies Hospital at Leazes Terrace 1966
Bed sitting room for mother and child
Audiovisual Centre, Newcastle University

TABLES

In the Text

From Page 132

INTRODUCTION

Six decades ago in 1954, Professor Sir James Calvert Spence, MC and Bar, MD, LLD (Durh), Hon. DSc, FRCP, died at the age of 62 years in Newcastle upon Tyne. He was one of the physicians of the first half of the 20th century who played an important part in the development of paediatrics and child health in the United Kingdom. Over the years, there have been several accounts of his achievements and tributes to his legacy In Newcastle and nationwide.[1 to 5, 7a and b to 10] Four publications stand out. There is a most valuable memoir by Lady Ursula Ridley who worked closely with him throughout most of the life of the Babies Hospital in Newcastle, which she described as "the essence of his achievement."[3] Sir John Charles, a close friend and former assistant medical officer of health for Newcastle and later Chief Medical Officer of Health for England, also wrote a memoir about his professional life in a memorial volume: 'The Purpose and Practice of Medicine.'[4] This contains a selection of Sir James' best known writings and lectures and a complete list of all his publications, including his clinical studies as well as those in the field of social paediatrics. Dr F.J.W. Miller wrote a concise biography.[5] He had his first encounter with Sir James (commonly known as J.C.) as a medical student in 1932. He eventually became a consultant paediatrician in Newcastle and in 1955, Reader in Social Paediatrics. He wrote that he was "captivated by his personality and 'outlook', and thereafter, except for the years 1942-5, worked with him until he died." Dr Miller was persuaded by J.C. to apply for the post of Senior Child Welfare Medical Officer in Newcastle in1938 and that year also joined the staff of the Babies Hospital as one of the honorary assistant physicians. He was a leading member of the Newcastle 1000 Families Study Group from the outset [18, 39, 40, 41] and also developed a special clinical expertise in childhood tuberculosis and the care of premature babies.[6] He initiated a home nursing care service when hospital services for the newborn were still poorly developed in Newcastle. This was the nucleus of the paediatric flying squad in later years.[38] He was awarded the Spence Medal in 1987 by the British Paediatric Association, the highest professional award in the United Kingdom for significant contributions to paediatrics and child health.

A comprehensive evaluation of J.C.'s legacy was published in 1975 by Professor Donald Court[10] who had worked with him as a Research Fellow from 1946 and succeeded him to the Chair of Child Health at Durham University (later the Newcastle University in 1963).

There are also two unpublished memoirs of personal recollections by Dr Miller[7a] and Dr E. Ellis,[8] who also had close links with J.C. as his registrar and first assistant and later became a consultant in Newcastle with a special interest in disability, notably cerebral palsy.

However, there has not yet emerged for publication a comprehensive study of J.C.'s clinical work at the Babies Hospital, where his pioneering contributions to paediatrics originated and his legacy took root. Also, there is as

1

yet no detailed account of J.C.'s legacy after the closure of the original Babies Hospital in 1945. He was no longer closely involved in the new Babies Hospital, which was established in 1948, when new clinical priorities emerged following the decline in infections. After his death, special hospital provisions for babies and infants with residential facilities for mothers, separate to the paediatric wards in the main hospitals in Newcastle, were still in place for a further 43 years to cater for the new challenges in paediatric practice.

It is possible now to make a new evaluation by analysing the detailed clinical data and commentaries in the Annual Reports of the Babies Hospital (1925 to 1945)[11] J.C. himself wrote the medical components, except for one year (1927) when he was away on a fellowship at John Hopkins Hospital in Baltimore, U.S.A., accompanied by his great friend Dr 'Jim' Bernard Shaw, with whom he spent a happy year there. Thereafter, there are bound volumes of Admission Records of a new Babies Hospital (1948-1976)[12] and reports from the Mother and Child (later Family) Unit at the Fleming Memorial Hospital for Sick Children (FMH) (1977-1985)[13] and the Family Unit at Newcastle General Hospital (NGH) (1987-1991)[14] These were the direct descendants of the Babies Hospital, where a similar ambience, nursing skills, accommodation for resident mothers and later partners, and expert paediatric care continued to meet the new challenges of vulnerable children. There is also an account of the history of the FMH (1887-1987).[15]

Sir James' legacy can thus be traced further objectively from the records of the hospital units that survived another half a century after he wrote the last medical report in 1945 of the first Babies Hospital.

His early life

Before describing the origins and evolution of his legacy, it is worth reflecting on his upbringing and life in medicine before he finally settled in Newcastle. This may shed some light on the roots of his vocation. This account is taken mainly from Sir John Charles' memoir.[4]

He was born in Amble, Northumberland, one of seven children. He had a settled, healthy and comfortable childhood. He read many books. His father was an architect and his grandfather a sea captain and ship builder in Northumberland. His medical background consisted of training at the University of Durham College of Medicine, where he graduated in1914 with second-class honours, six weeks before the outbreak of the First World War. He was commissioned in the Army to a Field Ambulance Unit and served with distinction in Gallipoli, Egypt, France and Belgium. He was awarded the Military Cross in 1917 and a Bar the following year for "his conspicuous gallantry and devotion to duty in proceeding to tend the wounded under heavy fire." His physical and mental state remained intact. On demobilisation, he came to Newcastle for six months as house physician to Dr Thomas Beattie at the Royal Victoria Infirmary (RVI). He then spent six months as Casualty Officer at Great Ormond Street Hospital (GOSH) in London. This was followed by a two year fellowship at St. Thomas Hospital in London with an interest in biochemical research. During this time, he had his first contact with the Medical Research Council (MRC). He was a member of a group from GOSH who investigated epidemic infantile diarrhoea, which was often fatal. He then returned permanently to Newcastle in 1922, when he was appointed medical registrar and chemical pathologist at the RVI. It was a time when the treatment of diabetes mellitus became a possibility and J.C. was in a position to take advantage of the opportunity with his knowledge of carbohydrate metabolism.

Although he had already taken an interest in childhood disease, he seemed set on a career in adult medicine. Notwithstanding any future commitment to the treatment of children's illnesses, he continued to see adults in private practice on a regular basis. This was the only way for a physician to earn a living in the north of England before the advent of the National Health Service in 1948. There was little opportunity for a private paediatric practice. Even after his appointment as a full honorary physician at the Royal Victoria Infirmary in 1939, his busy private consultant practice throughout the north east of England was almost entirely with adult patients, as private consultations regarding children were still infrequent. There are no distinctive indications in the early history of his life about the source and motivation that inspired him towards child health and paediatrics. What is evident is that he already showed in his early medical career an interest and aptitude for scientific research.[16, 17]

It is also likely that he realised very quickly that there was a dearth of knowledge about childhood disease during those early years of the 20th century. What is evident is that when he eventually settled in Newcastle, he came in contact with private individuals and doctors who had a passion and commitment to improve the wellbeing of children in a city, where poverty and poor social conditions had such a profound deleterious effect on the health of children and their families. The unfavourable environmental and social conditions during the first half of the 20th century are described in the Newcastle 1000 Families Study of 1947.[18] The high infant mortality rate compared with that in the rest of England and Wales[19] "furnished a grim index of social conditions" [Figure 1].

One of his acquaintances was Miss Greta Rowell, a friend who founded the West End Day Nursery in 1917. She was inspired by witnessing the plight of young children roaming the streets of Newcastle unaccompanied, whilst their mothers were employed in the munitions factories (Vickers Armstrong) during the daytime.[3]

He also came in contact with Dr Harold Kerr the medical officer of the city, who had already written about the extensive measures taken in Newcastle to alleviate the poor health and care of children by their families.[20] These began in the 1890s in response to a rise in infant mortality, which after a decline in the 1880s had risen to 193 per thousand births by 1899. There was also concern about a falling birth rate from 40 per thousand of the population during the later 1870s to 32 in 1894. These trends occurred nationally and were a considerable concern because the deficits, allied to the poor health of many adults in a diminishing population, were detrimental to the economic and social fabric of the nation. The Boer War in South Africa (1889-1902) had revealed the poor physical state of a significant proportion of army recruits. For example, in Manchester during 1899-1902 amongst 11000 men who had offered to enlist, three out of five were rejected as physically unfit and about a third of the remainder only just attained a moderate standard of physical fitness.[21]

The measures adopted in Newcastle as described by Dr Kerr included the appointment of female sanitary inspectors, a superintendent of midwives, trained nurses, health visitors and tuberculosis visiting nurses working from the dispensary. The Mothers and Babies Welcome Society founded in 1907 established seven welfare centres in the city, in which health visitors had a prominent role. Babies were weighed, mothers were taught child care and cheap food was provided for poor women through the later part of pregnancy and lactation. A crèche for working women was established with the collaboration of the Newcastle Public Health Department. Two doctors visited the welfare centres regularly, one for babies and another for the maternal welfare side. Dr Kerr decided to recruit 'active physicians' to conduct the welfare clinics and J.C. was one of his early appointees in 1923. This was his first contact with the City Health Department, a commitment he kept over the next 30 years. According to his friend Sir John Charles, this had "an incomparable effect on the development and future of social paediatrics in the country."[4] J.C. would thus have been aware of the local and national concerns about the health of the population at this early stage of his career as a children's physician. It was also an opportunity to gain experience of the lives of working class families, which he could hardly have acquired in any other way.

THE WEST END DAY NURSERY
33 WEST PARADE, NEWCASTLE-UPON-TYNE, 1918 - 1924

In 1923, at about the same time as his assignment to a child welfare clinic, J.C. accepted an appointment as Honorary Medical Officer to the West End Day Nursery in Newcastle. This was a pivotal moment in his medical career because it launched him into the field of paediatrics at a time when practical steps had already been taken to alleviate the ills and disadvantages of the poor, deprived children of Newcastle.

Miss Rowell had persuaded a wealthy anonymous donor (much later identified as Mr Frederick Milburn) to purchase the freehold of a suitable house and to provide £500 for equipment.[3] The West End Day Nursery opened in January 1918. She was the Honorary Secretary and Treasurer throughout its life. Dr Harold Kerr took a great interest in the nursery, one of the first of its kind in the country. During the year of J.C.'s appointment, he chaired the annual meeting of the Management Committee, which proposed the opening of a ward there for sick babies and infants under the age of three years. This is the first indication in Newcastle of the birth of a new kind of hospital for babies and the youngest children. Dr Kerr also indicated that he hoped to influence the City Council to give financial aid. This was forthcoming for the rest of the life of the Babies Hospital at West Parade and Blagdon Hall in Northumberland.

As a result of these events, several circumstances came together to arouse J.C.'s attention even before he started work in earnest at the nursery. In addition to his experience at the welfare clinic, he would have been aware of the poor physical condition of the children and the difficulties experienced by their mothers by reading the contents of the Annual Reports of the nursery dating back to 1919.[22] The medical data and commentaries were written by the Honorary Medical Officer, Dr H. L. Rutter MD, FRCS, DPH. He was a well-known local general practitioner, who continued his association with the day nursery until 1925, when he left for Birmingham on his appointment there as Regional Medical Officer under the Ministry of Health. His reports contain medical information and broad conclusions, which would have given J.C. an insight into the problems and adverse conditions that he was about to face. He would probably also have been aware of the discussions in 1923 of the reasons for opening an inpatient residential facility at the nursery. Therefore, much of the ground was already laid before his arrival for the development of a full-scale Babies Hospital and the later evolution of his ideas about the best way to care for babies and young children in a special hospital dedicated to this very young age group. It also paved the way for his initiatives in the field of social paediatrics.

A detailed analysis of the contents of the successive Annual Reports of the day nursery for 1919-1924, demonstrates the nature and extent of the information and insights that were already available to him before he started to work there.

In the Annual Report of 1919 for the year ending on the 31 December 1918, the object of the day nursery is defined:

"To provide a safe place where working mothers can leave their children in healthy surroundings with the knowledge that they will be properly cared for and well fed during the hours that they are compelled to leave them."

Dr Rutter declares his conclusions following the examination of 146 children attending the nursery:

"The frequency of improper feeding in the homes. Partly due to inexperience, but chiefly due to lack of honest care in preparation and giving of food. The lack of care in keeping children reasonably clean. The number of children in whom obvious diseases such as rickets are neglected and no medical advice sought."

He goes on to comment:

"It is not so much more knowledge that is needed by the mothers but the taking of the necessary trouble to apply the knowledge they have. Children need care and attention as well as love, and the first two necessitate a self denial that modern life and education fail to give."

Two years earlier in 1916, Dr T. E. Hill, the medical officer of health from nearby Durham County, had already commented on the chief cause of a high infant death rate in a nearby district. He attributed this not just to "especially bad conditions in regard to housing and overcrowding and lack of proper medical and nursing attentions for mothers and children," but firstly to "parental ignorance and physical inefficiency of mothers."[23]

In 1920, the object of the nursery was extended to cater for the needs of mothers in temporary distress or unable for domestic reasons to provide adequately for their children in their homes. Dr Rutter now goes on to record that he is:

"Convinced that most admissions occur because of ill-health of the child. Very few are in perfect health. Many have rickets, others are badly malnourished, have digestive troubles, are mentally below average and have physical defects such as club foot. For some children mothers give them little attention due to ignorance and neglect."

By now it was increasingly difficult to hold a balance between function as a nursery and a hospital on a small scale. In 1921, the 'broad conclusions' include the comment:

"Despite boasted advances of the twentieth century, if taking trouble, thought and self sacrifice are absent, children are bound to suffer."

He records that the nursery has three main aspects:

"Liberating the mother from anxiety of care during the day, when earning money or doing special work at home. The training of girls and young women in the care of babies and young children. This may be the most important function of the Day Nursery. Looking after and treating classes of children."

And finally the comment:

"A great deal is indirectly done to bring careless mothers to a greater degree of efficiency."

Dr Rutter had become convinced that most admissions occurred because of ill-health:

"When the child is ill, neighbours will not help."

His practice of writing perceptive commentaries may have encouraged J.C. to adopt the same methods. His extensive commentaries in later years will also be recorded verbatim in the present study, as they contribute so vividly to insights about his thoughts, teaching and actions.

Already during 1921, 14 probationers had received training at the nursery [Figure 2]. Eleven had been placed there by the Ministry of Labour. The training consisted of "practical experience in the feeding and management of infants and young children under 5 years, the washing of woollens etc., and the preparation of infant food." Each probationer had to make a set of infants' clothing. Lectures on first aid and infections were given by one of the honorary medical officers (Dr Mabel Campbell). The matron and the Honorary Secretary gave lectures on the care and management of children, nursery hygiene and elementary physiology. These educational activities anticipate the later training at the Babies Hospital. They resemble later day nursery nurse training.

That year, a number of children were in residence, three whose mothers were ill or had died. The following year, there were three children staying for one month. In January 1919, twins were admitted whose mother had to go into the Royal Victoria Infirmary for an operation. Then a further set of twins the following year, whose mother was ill with pneumonia; the family of five lived in one small room and one twin was already ill and had to be passed on to the Fleming Memorial Hospital for Sick Children. This is a potent example of the dreadful environmental conditions at that time in parts of Newcastle. Treatment was undertaken by Dr Rutter and the other honorary medical staff, Dr M. Campbell and Dr G. Muir.

In 1922, babies failing to thrive were put on humanised milk, anticipating the efficient arrangements later supervised by J.C. for a daily supply of human milk from known and certified sources as reported by him in 1925. Finally, in the important sixth report of 1924 (unfortunately the 1923 Annual Report could not be traced), Dr Rutter describes the transition from a day nursery to a nursing home. With the approval of the Ministry of Health, a ward was opened in October 1923 for infants suffering from 'marasmus'. J.C.'s name appears for the first time as one of the honorary medical officers, having begun to take part some time before May 1924.

The urgent need for a place where babies and infants with feeding difficulties could be scientifically looked after and treated had long been recognised. Local doctors had great difficulties in finding suitably trained nurses to care for these children at home and the main hospitals (RVI, NGH and FMH) were too full and preoccupied with seriously ill older children to cater for these cases. Also, special nursing skills were required. Between 9 October 1923 and 31 March 1924, ten children were admitted. Coincidentally with the change in the function of the nursery, there was a sharp decrease in the demand for day nursery places despite an intense publicity campaign [Table A]. This was associated with the massive post-war unemployment, which was particularly marked in the west end of the city now that the armaments industry reduced recruitment of women workers. Money was scarce and mothers stayed at home to care for their children. This eventually prompted the decision to close the Day Nursery. The case history of the first inpatient illustrates the problems that J.C. encountered when he started to work there:

"William P. was admitted on 9 October 1923 at the age of 16 weeks weighing only 9 lb 2½ oz. He was sent in by Dr Mabel Campbell from the Baby Welcome Clinic. There was some head retraction and he gave sharp cries suggestive of meningitis. He was ill-nourished and flabby. There was no vomiting or diarrhoea. He had been fed with Allen and Hanbury's Food for eight weeks. After admission his weight dropped nearly 2 lb to 7 lb 4 oz. He developed a pyrexia with septic spots and green stools. The pulse went up to about 170."

He gradually recovered and was discharged about 12 weeks later (aged 28 weeks) weighing 13 lb 7 oz, "looking a really healthy baby." The diagnosis remains obscure. The case histories of other inpatients are more straightforward:

"The baby was constantly vomiting. She weighed 10 lb 8½ oz (the age is not given). It was found that the mother was giving double strength milk. On humanised milk, the vomiting stopped immediately and seven weeks later she weighed 11 lb 9½ oz. It was found that even a slight increase in the feed (beyond one ounce) was upsetting her and she passed undigested food in the stools."

"Peggy B. Age 3 years had severe rickets. She improved slowly but steadily. Massage was included in her treatment."

Before discharge, the mothers attended the nursery for two days, "In order to carry on the same methods at home." Two children died. Both had meningitis and were moribund on admission. Dr Rutter comments:

8

"It is a question whether they should not have been sent straight out, but it was thought more humane not to send these dying children away, and with some regret we kept them in."

The final case history also demonstrates that under the label of 'marasmus', specific diagnoses were already being made:

"Betty S. was 1 year 9 months old. Her weight on admission was only 19 lb 15 oz (well below the 5th centile by present day standards). She was walking a little and had slight signs of rickets. Her stools contained more than 50% of fat and a diagnosis of coeliac disease was made. The treatment consisted of exclusion of all fat from the diet, limited carbohydrates and increased albumen. This was done by giving skimmed milk and adding casein in one form or another."

Dr Rutter adds:

"With Betty, it has been a long struggle week after week, month after month. Her weight went down by 8 lbs to 11 lb 15 oz, and she looked literally like skin and bones."

The child was still in the ward at the time of the Annual Report of 1924, five months after admission. The final comment is:

"The weight chart shows that she has regained some of the weight lost. If the child can possibly be kept alive, the disease often lasting months, gradually disappears."

The honorary physicians were most assiduous. They paid daily visits and J.C. also visited frequently. Dr Rutter states that on the opening of the ward:

"Daily and often more frequent medical visits were required, but your medical staff have, with pleasure, visited as often as necessary."

It is already clear at this early stage of J.C.'s involvement that a detailed, carefully thought out nursing and medical care programme had been established with close amicable collaboration between all the staff, a sound example and basis for J.C.'s later developments at the Babies Hospital.

9

Table A. The West End Day Nursery. 1918-1924

	1919	1920	1921	1923	1924
Attendances in previous year	4305	4293	5307	4025	2764
Opening hours	0745 - 1900	0700 - 1900	0700 – 1900	not	recorded
Charges/day *	9 pence	6 pence	9 pence	not	recorded
Comments	Outbreaks of measles and cases of bronchitis, diarrhoea. Rickets in many. 4 had massage (2 with malnutrition, 1 rickets, 1 clubfoot)	Few infections. 4 whooping cough, 2 chicken pox, 1 mumps. Masseuse was treating 'backward' children.	No infectious diseases but many sore throats. Admissions of children because 5 mothers unwell or had died (3 became residents).3 admitted for massage only	7 cases of whooping cough. 2 chicken pox. Many winter colds. Babies failing to thrive put on humanised milk. 3 children resident for 1 month.	Closed in April 1923 for 2 weeks because of measles. 50% of children examined had large tonsils. 4 with mild chicken pox. A ward opened in October. 10 inpatients-infants with failure to thrive, marasmus, rickets and feeding difficulties.

* During 1921, the average wages in agriculture and forestry were of the order of 24 shillings per week, for miners 48s, in manufacturing 36s, for local government civil servants 48s, for the military 37s and 84s for those in insurance, banking and finance.[135] Women were often receiving a lot less - often less than half that of the men. The salary of the first matron of the West End Day Nursery, who was a State Registered Nurse, was £50 a year 'resident with laundry and uniform allowance of £4'. The assistant matron received £30.[3]

THE BABIES NURSERY AND MOTHERCRAFT CENTRE
(1924 – 1925)
AT 33 WEST PARADE, NEWCASTLE-UPON TYNE

The new name signifies the change in function from a day nursery to an inpatient hospital facility. An inspector from the Ministry of Health had indicated that there was then no further need for day nurseries. It finally closed on 13 September 1924. During the year between 1 April 1924 and 31 March 1925, 53 infants were admitted as inpatients. They were referred by doctors in private practice, the Newcastle Maternity and Infant Welfare Department, the Citizens Service Society, the Diocesan Rescue Workers and the Durham County Maternity Infant Welfare Office. This is already a relatively wide range of sources of referral from beyond Newcastle. It indicates the urgent need for this kind of service in the north east of England.

Table B. The Annual Medical Report. 1925
Diagnoses on Admission

Marasmus	27
Prematurity	2
Rickets	12
Tetany	2
Pyloric stenosis	1
Coeliac disease	1
Severe vomiting	1
Tuberculosis	4
No appreciable disease	3
Total Number	53

In July 1924, J.C. accepted the position of Honorary Consulting Physician. He was now the chief physician at the Babies Nursery. Within a few months of his arrival, he assumed leadership as chairman of the medical and surgical staff to develop the service. Just after his promotion, he was due to visit the Ministry of Health in London in order to discuss the kind of services offered at the West End Babies Nursery.[3]

11

The medical report for 1925 is not signed, but has all the characteristics of J.C.'s later reports from the Babies Hospital. This applies in particular to the tabulation of diseases, shown in Table B, above.

The ages of the inpatients are not given, but in contrast to most of the children attending the day nursery, they are now referred to as 'infants', so that the majority were probably under the age of 1 year. Thirty-nine (73.5%) were discharged, cured or greatly improved. Three were transferred to other hospitals. Three were taken out unimproved and eight (15%) died. Compared to similar hospitals in the country, it is recorded in the report that this was a low mortality and a high recovery rate.

The commentary includes an account of the principles of treatment for the purpose of training and management. The Truby King methods of the Mothercraft Society at Cromwell House in London were in use.[25] 'Breast fed was best fed', but when this failed, a scientifically balanced milk was substituted. The rules were rigid with strict adherence to four-hourly feeding and test weighing at every feed to prevent over-feeding. Such a rigid regime frustrated attempts to persevere with breastfeeding and particularly its re-establishment after illness. It was discontinued after 1925, as it did not take account of the functional, physiological aspects of breast milk production. One of the chief advantages available to treat infants with marasmus was a plentiful daily supply of human milk from known and certified sources. In all cases, the sources of the milk were under supervision and medically examined and each supply was collected and conveyed to the nursery with suitable precautions. The method and organisation of the collection of human milk was, as far as is known, a new and unique step in England. It was pointed out:

"The treatment of marasmus requires great nursing care and highly technical tasks of nursing. It is one of the most difficult tasks in nursing."

There is an important comment in relation to the 12 children with rickets:

"It is a preventable and curable disease."

The incidence was declining rapidly in the south of England, but remained high in Newcastle and other northern industrial towns. This was very noticeable during the spring months of 1925 following a particularly long sunless autumn and winter.

Outpatient sessions were started, two afternoons a week, for consultations and the examination of children for admission. Mothers came regularly for help and support for breastfeeding and infants arrived for sunray treatment of rickets by means of a mercury vapour lamp. This was the first piece of equipment that J.C. persuaded the Management Committee to purchase in 1926 [Figures 3a and 3b]. The cost was met by an anonymous donor.

The year was punctuated by periods of rapid re-organisation and reconstruction. The nursery was then fully equipped for a modern babies and infants hospital. J.C. was already looking to the future, anticipating a rapid and sharp increase in demand as there were no similar hospital provisions in the

12

north east of England. That year on his recommendation, an Honorary Consultant Surgeon, Mr F.C. Pybus, MD (Durh), FRCS, was appointed.

The overwhelming impression on a reading of this report from 1925 is of a well organised, dynamic hospital with a rational, scientific, forward looking approach and highly skilled nursing staff able to care for some of the most severely malnourished and ill babies and infants. Also, a most assiduous medical staff working in close, amicable collaboration with the nurses and a strongly supportive management committee that worked to finance and promote the nursery – a recipe for J.C.'s future development of a pioneering hospital service for sick babies and infants for Newcastle and the northern region.

THE BABIES HOSPITAL AND MOTHERCRAFT CENTRE
1 APRIL 1925 to 31 MARCH 1937
AT 33 WEST PARADE, NEWCASTLE-UPON-TYNE

After 1925, the Babies Nursery became a well-established hospital. This is reflected in the change of name to "The Babies Hospital and Mothercraft Centre." [Figure 4] The majority of the inpatients were under the age of 12 months [Table 1; Appendix 1]. In 1930, a verandah was added to the hospital, which made it possible to increase the proportion of children aged over 12 months to 39%. This was used for the open-air treatment of rickets, which occurred frequently around the age of 12 months, and for infants with tuberculosis. By 1936, the proportion of infants under the age of 3 months had settled to about one half (53%) with only about a quarter (22%) over the age of 12 months. From the outset, the hospital catered primarily for children under the age of 3 years.

Soon after J.C. assumed the leadership at the hospital, there are early indications of his authority. His nomination as an honorary consultant was also intended by the Committee of Management to elevate his status shortly before he was due to visit the Ministry of Health in London to discuss the new Babies Hospital, as there were no other similar hospital provisions in the north east of England. The appointment, on his recommendation, of Mr F. C. Pybus, was a real coup for the hospital. He was a local graduate with a first class honours degree and a reputation as an outstanding surgeon.[26] He retired in 1953 and became Emeritus Professor of Surgery in the University of Durham.

J.C. continued to develop friendly collaboration with the Management Committee chaired by Lady Ridley. By 1937, the Annual Report records:

"The development of the hospital's work is marked by a unity of purpose and spirit of harmony to which the administrative staff, the Medical Staff and the Nursing Staff all contribute."

Mothers in residence

This is for many the outstanding contribution of J.C. to the care of children in hospital. The insights gained from this experience and the benefits that followed led eventually to a significant increase of understanding by the medical profession and the public of mother and child attachment and the needs of young children. From a low number of nine (10%) out of 86 in 1925, 70 (21%) out of 339 were admitted with their mothers in 1936 (Table 1).

For the first time in 1925, one room of the hospital had been set aside for a mother to establish breastfeeding. One of the earliest cases illustrates the benefits:

14

"A very wasted infant, who had weighed 6½ lbs at birth, only weighed 5 lbs at the age of 6 weeks. He had been artificially fed with a variety of foods from the bottle. Breast feeding was successfully established for the first time after two weeks. He gained 2 lbs during the first month in Hospital and at the age of 6 months at home, he was fully breast fed and his weight was normal."

In 1928, two rooms were made available. Eleven mothers came in, six for re-establishing breastfeeding in infants who:

"Had been unnecessarily weaned and were wasting in consequence,"

and five in order to maintain breastfeeding in infants with intercurrent illnesses. All were successful. In 1931, J.C. commented:

"Judging from the trend of the work, it appears that the chief demand in the immediate future will be for increased accommodation for mothers so that they can be admitted and kept in hospital with their infants when the continuation of breast feeding demands it."

He was confirming the increase in the criteria for admission. Eight rooms became available in 1931 as a result of an extension following the purchase of a house next door.

During the two years from 1930-1931, 47 mothers came into residence with infants requiring an operation. Nearly all had pyloric stenosis. In 1936, J.C. wrote:

"In former years it was our custom to admit mothers only when it was necessary for them to maintain breast feeding. In the past year, we have extended this plan and admitted mothers whenever the nature of their infant's illness demanded her care and nursing. We are convinced of the success of this plan. With the cooperation of matron and the nursing staff it works smoothly. It solves many of the hitherto insuperable difficulties of the satisfactory nursing of sick infants in Hospital and we look forward to further developments of this plan so as to make it the central feature of our nursing organisation in the future. No breast fed infant has died following an operation for the sixth year in succession."

J.C. states:

"Its value will be realised from the fact that it is used chiefly in the care of critically ill infants requiring an operation. Experience shows that the best results are obtained by putting the infants in sole charge of one person throughout its stay in hospital. It is a satisfactory solution of the problem for the mother to undertake this duty under the supervision and instruction of a nursing sister."

He ends by reiterating:

15

"We aim still further development of this plan until we are able to accommodate whenever necessary each mother with her sick infant in their own single room."

Mothers eagerly welcomed the practice. Lady Ridley in her memoir[3] writes:

"It was remarkable how many of them managed to find substitutes at home, and how eagerly the opportunity was seized, mothers often turning up at outpatients with a suitcase even before they knew their child was admitted."

The single rooms were made as comfortable and homely as possible [Figure 5]. About 20 years later in the Charles West Lecture at the Royal College of Physicians of London, entitled 'The Care of Children in Hospitals', J.C. summed up the benefits.[27] It is the most comprehensive expression of his views and is recorded here in full:

"The mother lives in the same room as her child. She needs little or no off-duty time, because the sleep requirements of a mother fall near to zero when the child is acutely ill. She feeds the child; she tends the child; she keeps it in its most comfortable posture, whether on its pillow or her knee. The sister and nurse are at hand to help and administer treatment to the child. The advantages of the system are fourfold. It is an advantage to the child. It is an advantage to the mother, for to have undergone this experience and to have felt that she has been responsible for her own child's recovery establishes a relationship with her child and confidence in herself which bodes well for their future. It is an advantage to the nurses, who learn much by contact with the best of these women, not only about the handling of a child but about life itself. It is an advantage to the other children in the ward, for whose care more nursing time is liberated. In teaching hospitals, it is of further advantage to the students, who gain practical experiences of the form of nursing they will depend on in their practices and learn to recognise the anxieties and courage which bind the mothers to their children during their illness; a lesson which fosters the courtesy on which the practice of medicine depends. I advocate this method of nursing, not on sentimental grounds but on the practical grounds of efficiency and necessity. Apart from all other reasons, the shortage of nurses will impose the method on us in the future."

In every Annual Report, he acknowledges the extent to which the work of the hospital depends on the skill and devotion of matron and the nursing staff. In 1936, he writes that the work:

"Is carried out in a manner which gives the Hospital the atmosphere of a home rather than an institution, and this earns the gratitude both of the Staff and the patients."

The information recorded in the Annual Reports[11]

In order to underpin an understanding of the evolving work of the hospital throughout its life from 1925 to1945 and the extent of J.C.'s involvement, the data in these reports is collated in Tables 1 to 9 and Figures 6, 11, 13 and 18. These records are complemented by J.C.'s regular commentaries. As in the case of his comments relating to mothers in residence, these are recorded verbatim because they provide such a vivid insight into his powers of observation and analysis, as well as his ability to communicate in simple, non-technical language. Appendix 2 includes the example of a Medical Report from 1931-32.

There are two separate discrepancies in the recorded data (Tables 5a and 5b). For six years from 1931 to 1936, the data for the total number of recorded diagnoses does not match the number of new admissions recorded during those years. There is a shortfall of the order of 21% (range 17-30%). The reason is that only the 'commonest', 'most important' or 'chief' diagnoses are recorded. It is likely that the shortfall occurred in the number of different medical disorders recorded (other than infections). Table 2 shows that during those years, infections and pyloric stenosis continued to be recorded consistently in relatively high numbers and a large number of infants with congenital malformations consisting mainly of infants with hare lip and cleft palate were treated. The less numerous diagnoses of tuberculosis, rickets and Pink Disease continued at about the same level as in previous years.

There is further evidence for this conclusion. A rise in the number of 'miscellaneous medical diagnoses' had occurred before 1931 [Table 2] and resumed after 1936 [Table 6]. During the period of the deficit there was no decrease in the total number of admissions; indeed the number increased and remained at a steady level right up to the outbreak of the war in 1939 [Tables 1 and 4]. In addition, J.C. had reported an increase in the number of medical diagnoses during 1931, which is confirmed by the list of conditions recorded at postmortem that year. Infants with renal disease, chronic chest conditions and convulsions were noted. None of these conditions are recorded in the Annual Reports during the years of the deficits, nor were any under the label of "miscellaneous medical conditions", which were otherwise recorded every year before 1931 and after 1936. There is thus a compelling case for the correction of the data in Figure 6 of the number of "miscellaneous medical conditions" encountered during those years. This has been done.

The other inconsistency is the lack of precision before 1936 in the identification of infants with hare lip and cleft palate. These two conditions were included amongst the total number of congenital malformations recorded during those years. Throughout the life of the Babies Hospital up to 1945, infants with congenital malformations were seldom admitted unless they required an operation and few were carried out other than for hare lip and cleft palate. For example, in 1933 there were only four amongst 45 cases of congenital disorders. It is therefore safe to assume that, before 1936, most admissions recorded as congenital malformations consisted of infants for operation on hare lip and cleft palate. This conclusion is reinforced by the comments in the surgical

17

section of the Annual Reports, which record an increasing number at earlier ages of successful operations for these conditions.

For all these reasons, Figure 6 has been drawn to clarify these discrepancies. The conclusion is that the number of diagnoses of 'miscellaneous medical conditions' and operations for pyloric stenosis, hare lip and cleft palate continued at a high level comparable to that of infections during 1931 to 1936.

The changing pattern of diagnoses, 1924-1936 [Figure 6]

During the first 12 years of the hospital, there were some striking changes. Marasmus gave way to medical and surgical disorders. Infections and infants with pyloric stenosis, hare lip and cleft palate dominated. By 1936, these two surgical categories accounted for nearly a quarter of all the admissions that year. The criteria for admission were necessarily strict because of the persistent and considerable shortage of accommodation. Only the most seriously ill children were considered for admission from amongst those with infections. Some moribund children, who died within a day or so, were admitted in the hope that something might be done for them. The relatively high mortality of up to about 20% each year may be partly explained by these considerations. Infants requiring an operation for pyloric stenosis, hare lip and cleft palate were given priority because, otherwise, many were likely to have died at home. If the operation was a success, and most of them did eventually survive, a complete cure was achieved. Skilled nursing and medical care as well as the maintenance of breastfeeding were important contributions to these successes.

Marasmus

At the outset this was the predominant diagnosis [Figures 6 and 7]. In 1926, when there was a peak in the number of these admissions - 55 cases representing 54% of all new admissions (Table 2) - J.C. defined 'marasmus' as a term:

"Which is applied to so large a proportion of the cases as a convenient one to use for the large group of infants suffering from malnutrition of ill-defined origin. Where definite organic disease is detectable, the term is inadmissible, but it is just in this type of case that the careful feeding and nursing only to be obtained in a Hospital such as this, are of outstanding importance. Many of these infants could not be reared under home conditions"

The yearly numbers declined, but in 1929 J.C. was still commenting:

"It is one of the problems of disease in infancy that usually produced marked wasting and malnutrition, and it is for this that most cases are admitted. In such cases, the question of some underlying or latent disease has to be considered."

18

A plot on a modern centile chart (from the 1970s) of the weights on admission during 1926 illustrates the wasting in male infants under the age of 1 year [Figure 8].

The same applied equally to female infants. As the number of infants with marasmus declined, a greater number of specific medical diseases and infections were identified. Thus in 1930, there were 7 pyelonephritis, 5 anaemia, 9 Pink Disease, 3 meningitis, 2 paratyphoid fever and 21 with bronchopneumonia or pneumonia. The last record of marasmus appears in the 7th Annual Report of 1931, when there were only 13 (6%) out of the 162 diagnoses recorded that year.

Acute infections

There is a steep rise in the number of acute infections. In 1926, there were only seven (7%) out of a total of 102 new admissions; ten years later in 1936, there were 103 (30%) recorded in 339 new admissions. J.C. comments repeatedly on the aetiology, the factors contributing to the high prevalence and the consequences.

A diagnosis of 'general sepsis and its effects' is first recorded in 1930, rising from 20 cases that year to 46 in 1936. In 1932, he reports the good news of a steady decline of infective gastro-enteritis in recent years. On the other hand, he notes a relative increase in diseases of the lungs especially infective bronchopneumonia:

"It is significant that whereas pneumonia is a frequent cause of death in ill-nourished or improperly fed children, it is rarely fatal amongst those who are well-nourished."

In the preceding year, there had been 12 deaths of infants with bronchopneumonia, which together with the nine cases of gastro-enteritis accounted for about 44% of the deaths that year. This prompted him to write:

"This reveals the great importance of an adequate and balanced diet in maintaining resistance to diseases. On this point, the experience of the medical staff is that the majority of the children from the towns and country districts are not undernourished but improperly fed, due mainly to the excessive amount of cereal and bread which is provided in their diets. It is a danger that the people in the country eat too much wheat food to the exclusion of root vegetables."

In 1934, J.C. reported that they had been dealing with and studying the effects of septicaemia and septic infections in newborn infants. He concludes:

"It is now more clearly recognised that septic infections which are harmless to older children or adults may be a potent cause of death in young infants."

19

This is the first record in the Annual Reports of the realisation that infections were such a dominant factor in the high mortality and morbidity of babies and infants. In 1937, he notes explicitly:

"It is probable that the relatively high infant mortality which persists in Newcastle and the surrounding area is largely accounted for in this manner."

By now it may be inferred that these conclusions will have set in train a course of events that a few years later led J.C. to undertake the Infant Mortality Survey with Dr F.J.W. Miller[28] and later the "1000 Families Study in Newcastle upon Tyne."[18] These confirmed the overwhelming contribution of infections to the mortality and morbidity of the young children of the city during that era.

Furthermore, from his extensive experience of the circumstances of the families that came to the hospital, he came very soon to an understanding of the importance of some of the adverse family and social-environmental factors that affected their health and welfare. In 1932, he comments:

"With many infants coming to the Hospital from different towns and districts, it has been possible to assess the great variation in the mothercraft of the women, that is their capacity to care for and look after their infants. It is evident that the mothercraft of the urban mother is usually much below that of the mother from the outlying districts. It is particularly noticeable that the women from the Northumbrian villages, wives of miners and workers, inherit and maintain that capacity in a high degree. They are well endowed with shrewd common sense and sagacity which makes good mothers of them."

The persistent shortage of accommodation

This is a recurrent theme throughout the life of the hospital. In 1926, J.C. wrote:

"The question can be solved only by raising public interest in the matter, and as a preliminary to this, it requires to be realised how entirely fallacious is the argument that hospital treatment of sick and wasting infants is fostering the survival of the unfit. Those countries that have the most ample provision for the hospital treatment of children have the highest level of health and fitness in their adult peoples."

At times, the shortage of cots was so severe that infants had to be discharged sooner than the staff would have wished, in order to make room for urgent cases. J.C. went on to write:

"This raises the problem of the great lack of beds for the inpatient hospital treatment of infants in Newcastle. The town serves as a hospital centre for a very wide area, and during the year, cases have been admitted to our own hospital from all the Northern Counties. On this basis, there ought to be available for treatment of general medical diseases of infants more than three times the accommodation that is at present provided in the various institutions. As it is, this hospital although small, provides more than half the present available accommodation. One result of this lack is that many infants are admitted at the late stage of disease when much more might have effectively been done if earlier admission had been possible."

By 1936, after two adjacent houses had been bought, there were 36 beds including an eight bedded ward and verandah for infants with tuberculosis and rickets.

Surgery [Table 9]

This was an important component of the inpatient service of the hospital. By 1935, 77 operations were done that year. The great success of the service was dependent not only on the skill of the surgeons, the anaesthetists and the nursing staff, but also the close involvement of the medical staff in pre- and post-operative care. J.C. noted in 1933:

"We are glad to report that progress continues in solving the problems of the pre-operative care of these cases. This is effected mainly as a result of the system of cooperation and conference amongst members of the staff which prevails in the Hospital."

From the outset, the hospital specialised in the operative care of three conditions, pyloric stenosis and hare lip and cleft palate, which were commonly complicated by severe malnutrition and wasting. They were often fatal when admission was delayed and they required just the kind of expert nursing skills available at the hospital and virtually nowhere else in the northern districts.

The first operation was performed in 1925 on an infant with pyloric stenosis. It is recorded that as:

"It did not do very well, the second case was sent to the RVI for operation, returning to the Babies Hospital a few days later."

Over the next four years, this condition was treated medically. Most were seriously ill and wasted on admission and took many weeks to improve. J.C. commented that it makes:

"Supreme demands on nursing skills."

The first consistent record of operations on pyloric stenosis is in the medical report for 1929. J.C. notes:

"Progress has been made in the earlier recognition of the pyloric cases and the advances in the methods of surgical treatment."

Some congenital deformities, especially hare lip and cleft palate, were also operated on. It is the latter that soon became the particular speciality of the hospital, following the appointment in 1928 of Mr W.E.M. Wardill as Honorary Surgeon. Writing further about pyloric stenosis, J.C. comments:

"It is a disease which can be completely and speedily cured when promptly treated."

Two years earlier, he had pointed out:

"This disease is an example of the necessity of exact and early diagnosis, for if not recognised it is uniformly fatal."

These comments explain the principal reason for the steep increase in the number of infants with pyloric stenosis treated in the hospital. The same applies to infants with hare lip and cleft palate, with the added incentive that the hospital was acquiring a national reputation for the successful operative treatment of these conditions.

In 1932, 40 infants with pyloric stenosis had an operation with seven (17.5%) deaths and J.C. comments:

"It accounts for a good deal of the nutritional disorders and wasting of infants."

He goes on to note:

"Twenty years ago it was rarely recognised; ten years ago it was not commonly diagnosed; of late the nature of the disease has become well known on account of the work done in voluntary hospitals."

He too should be given credit for educating doctors during his regular lectures and ward rounds and in promoting the achievements of the Babies Hospital. As in all of his medical reports, he praises and thanks the nursing staff:

"We have to acknowledge how great a benefit has been derived from the special nursing arrangements which have been made in our hospital for the individual care and treatment of these infants before and after operation."

The first independent surgical report appears in the 8th Annual Report of 1 April 1931 to 31 March 1932. It is unsigned but was probably written by Mr Wardill, who was responsible for all future surgical reports until the outbreak of the Second World War in 1939. It is recorded that:

"It is noticeable that a fair proportion of the infants are admitted to hospital in an extreme state of emaciation, and cannot be regarded as good surgical risks; particularly does this apply in the case of infants above the age of 6 weeks. The cause for this probably lies in the fact that, owing to the present industrial depression, parents are slow to seek the advice of their doctors, and from this case alone there is likely to be a continuance of this mortality."

By 1936, the outcome of operations for pyloric stenosis had greatly improved. Compared with a mortality of 50% in 1930, it was down to less than 4%, one of the lowest mortality recorded nationwide during that era. 26 out of 27 infants admitted that year had an operation with one death. It was Mr Wardill now who acknowledged:

"The improvement in the figures is to be attributed to earlier diagnosis by outside doctors, and the increased experience of the Nursing and Medical Staff of the Babies Hospital."

Following the first record of operations for hare lip in 1929, the surgery for this condition and for cleft palate increased. In 1932, a special outpatient follow-up clinic for these malformations was established. A year later in 1933, Mr Wardill reports:

"Considerable advances have been made owing to the perfection of endotracheal methods by Dr W.J. Phillips. Owing to this work it is now possible to carry on an operation in the most deliberate fashion and absolutely consistent with safety. This part of the work has been rendered all the more easy by the cooperation of the Medical Staff, the Matron and the Nurses."

A year later in 1934, operations for cleft palate were done at an earlier age. Mr Wardill acknowledged:

"The assistance of Dr Spence, Dr Ogilvie and Dr Wright [Honorary Assistant Physicians] has succeeded in eliminating cases which would otherwise have been regarded as bad surgical risks. There has been no mortality (to date) from this operation."

Excellent results were also recorded from the special outpatient follow-up clinic set up in 1932 [Figure 9]. There was now "a large proportion in which none of the usual defects of speech are observable."

One of the earliest speech therapists, Miss (later Dr) Muriel Morley, who was associated with this outpatient clinic from 1933, became the leading speech therapist of the United Newcastle Hospitals and a founding member of the Newcastle University Department of Speech and Language Studies. This began with the establishment of a Sub-Department of Speech from the 1st April 1959 in the Department of Child Health, with the strong support of Professor Court.[31a] She was also a leading member of a special clinic introduced by Professor Court in 1949 for the assessment and treatment of speech and language disorders in young children. Dr Morley wrote two classic books based on her work at the Babies Hospital. In 'Cleft Palate and Speech' (1945)[29], she paid tribute to the skills of Mr Wardill and Miss Cummings, matron at the Babies Hospital, who adopted special methods of artificial feeding in cases of cleft palate.

In 'The Development and Disorders of Speech in Childhood' (1957)[30], she drew on her extensive clinical experience at the Babies Hospital which later extended to the homes, schools and relevant institutions of the local community. She was passionate about the personal and social importance of speech and the promotion of its academic study.[31b] The special clinic of 1932 at the hospital was thus the forerunner of the pioneering University Department of Speech and Language and the specialist services for children in Newcastle.[31a] It was the first University in the United Kingdom to award a degree in Speech and Language Therapy in 1967.[31b]

In 1935, Dr Philip Ayre (Honorary Anaesthetist) devised a T tube for operations on cleft palate, which "far exceeds in safety and utility anything that has hitherto been tried." By 1936, there were 26 operations for hare lip with one death and 21 for cleft palate, also with one death "attributed entirely to causes beyond our control."

By this time, the hospital's successful treatment of cleft palate was attracting national and international attention. A relatively small number of other operations were carried out over the years. For example, in 1933 there were: one abscess of neck, two hernias, one intestinal obstruction, one spina bifida and one for phimosis.

Under J.C.'s leadership, the close collaboration between physicians, surgeons and nursing staff led to the rapid expansion and improvements in the surgical service. As so many of the infants were wasted and in poor physical condition, the close involvement of the physicians and the special skills of the nursing staff were always vital components of pre-and post-operative care. It is not generally known that a significant proportion of the inpatient services of the Babies Hospital was eventually devoted to the treatment of pyloric stenosis, hare lip and cleft palate. From the first operations in 1929 to 1935, approximately one-fifth of all inpatients at the hospital had treatment for these conditions; by 1936 to 1944, the proportion had risen to one-third of all admissions.

Specific diagnoses

As the number of diagnoses of marasmus declined, more specific medical conditions were identified. By 1930, these included chronic chest diseases, neonatal disorders, anaemia, and Pink Disease. The new diagnosis of pyelonephritis is a good example. It was often fatal - in 1929, eight out of 12 died.

Already in 1926, J.C. had acquired a small laboratory adjacent to the outpatient clinic. Clinical assistants were appointed to undertake practical tasks and recording. There were five in 1927 and a variable number in later years.

Feeding difficulties

In 1935-1936, feeding difficulties are recorded. These must have been severe, probably with much wasting:

"With simple feeding disorders an attempt has been made to deal with these simply as out-patients when the home conditions have been satisfactory. Where loss of weight has been found to be severe."

J.C. had commented in 1930:

"Due to improper or inadequate feeding these measures have usually been sufficient. Moreover, it is the type of case which is well provided for in the town and certain other districts where there are welfare clinics."

Dyspepsia

This condition was sometimes recorded in association with marasmus. In 1933-1936, it is recorded on its own. A term unfamiliar in paediatric practice today, it derives from the Greek meaning 'bad-cooking' and is defined in the Oxford Compact Dictionary as:

"A disorder of the digestive organs, especially the stomach, weakness, wasting, loss of appetite and depression of spirits."

Pink Disease (Erythroedema)

J.C. first recorded this illness in 1926. He notes four years later:

"Amongst the patients seen and treated at the hospital there have been many cases of a peculiar disease known as Pink Disease, which appears to be on an increase in the community and of which more cases have been reported from this district than from any other part of the country. It is a disease peculiar to infancy, with a high mortality, and so far the cause has not been discovered. The medical staff is continuing to devote attention to the problem. Only the severest cases have been admitted to hospital and opportunity has been able to demonstrate that it is not due to any deficiency of diet and that it is not a transmissible infective disease."

By 1933, more than 100 affected infants had been seen at the hospital and 66 were admitted for inpatient treatment between 1926 and 1936. Twelve (18%) died. Fourteen years later in 1950, J.C. published a paper describing his experience of 404 cases.[4a] He noted the 'inexplicable misery' of the condition, with as yet no cause found. He concluded that the best treatment is:

"The solacing, nursing and comforting by a careful mother with such sedation as may be necessary."

The cause was finally determined in 1954.[32] It was due to poisoning by mercury in teething powders and also occurred in great numbers in other parts of the country.

It is of historical interest that there was such a prolonged delay before the connection was made. After 1948, J.C. considered the possibility of mercury poisoning, but concluded that the evidence was inconclusive. Excessive amounts of mercury were found in the urine of infants with Pink Disease. However, it was not present in all of them and he believed that many did not have any contact with it.[32]

It has been suggested that, nationwide, the delay in establishing a cause was related to the medical and social context of those years. Doctors on the whole did not have "a mental image of poisoning as a cause of disease in childhood."[32] They were not in the habit of enquiring about the contents of medicines given by mothers on their own initiative and did not take account of these in assessing causes. The emphasis was on infections (especially viruses) and defective nutrition. J.C. and his colleagues had excluded transmittable disease and dietary deficiency during the early 1930s. In 1938, he wrote:

"Many observers have remarked that it is more likely to occur in the children of well-cared for families than those of poverty-stricken families; further, in so many instances, the infant diet had been reinforced by orange juice, cod-liver oil, marmite and other foods rich in vitamins that the possibility that it is a disease of overnutrition must be considered."[32]

In addition and more generally, it is also suggested:

"Speculation about its cause and cure was limited and misled by contemporary fashion in medical thinking about the nature of disease, by a concentration on known and currently fashionable causes of disease and by a lack of interest in both the general nature of aetiology of disease and in the possible influence of infant life and care."

These observations do not apply to J.C., who was singularly intent on establishing a cause of illness in order to provide effective remedies on the basis of objective evidence. Nevertheless, there are no recorded initiatives by him to investigate the contents of teething powders or any other medicines acquired by parents. It was not until after 1954, when mercury was withdrawn from teething powder voluntarily by manufacturers because of adverse publicity about the dangers of mercury ingestion generally, that Pink Disease in infants disappeared suddenly and the connection was universally accepted.

Rickets

Infants with severe rickets continued to be admitted. Treatment consisted of an appropriate diet, plenty of fresh air, artificial sunlight by means of a mercury vapour lamp and massage. Two honorary masseuses were engaged. Milder cases were treated as outpatients. In 1933, J.C. published the results of a controlled trial of the antirachitic activity of calciferol. This was done at the request of the Therapeutic Trials Committee of the Medical Research Council and demonstrated a significant benefit.[33] Sir John Charles in his memoir of 1960,[4] commented that it:

"Was one of the earliest and conclusive of a now long series of controlled trials. It established Spence's reputation as a clear-eyed investigator in the difficult fields where clinical acumen and scientific precision have need to walk hand in hand."

Although treatment with calciferol is not recorded, it is likely to have been prescribed at the hospital. There is no record of specific drug treatment of any kind in the Annual Reports of the Babies Hospital. There was no dispensing in the outpatient clinic; the drugs that were recommended had to be obtained by the parents from the children's family doctors.

Tuberculosis

This disease was a potent cause of illness in the community and infants were admitted persistently over the years, especially when home conditions were unsatisfactory for adequate care. There are repeated commentaries by J.C. in the Annual Reports as the nature, the progress of the disease and the most appropriate care were identified. In 1926, J.C. notes:

"The cases of tuberculosis are of special interest in view of the medical and social problems involved. It is now widely recognised that tuberculosis in infancy is fairly common, although it may exist in forms difficult to recognise without prolonged observation and investigation. Moreover, the source of infection in these cases is usually some accidental contact with an adult suffering from the disease. We have been able to prove this in some of our cases."

He goes on that year to record the discovery of BCG and the provisions that have to be made to treat the disease:

"Certain recent discoveries have been made in France which appear to promise that, a new method of preventative treatment may shortly be available for children who stand in danger of exposure to infection. This will mark a great advance in the control of the disease, and it renders it important that we should continue to provide all available accommodation for the treatment and study of these cases."

He highlighted repeatedly the lack of appropriate convalescent facilities in the northern districts, especially as many homes were not found to be satisfactory when the child was ready for discharge from the hospital. For this reason, a verandahh was built by 1931 on the south side of the hospital to accommodate up to six cots for convalescent cases [Figure 10]. This was paid for by the 'Mile of Pennies' scheme initiated by Miss D. Richardson, a member of the Hospital House Committee. The 1935 report notes that the hospital is:

27

"Forced to undertake this work owing to lack of provision elsewhere for the special treatment of tuberculosis in infants under the age of three."

Studies of the disease continued and in 1932, he published a paper with the case histories of two infants aged 6 and 7 months and a toddler of 5 years.[34a] They had what he termed "benign tuberculous infiltration of the lung" (epituberculosis). The disease was characterised by failure to thrive, extensive consolidation of the lung with relatively slight illness and a strongly positive tuberculin test. After several months in hospital, the consolidation receded and all recovered. In the light of more definitive diagnoses in marasmic infants, it is of interest that the 7 month old infant was brought to the hospital in 1931 for advice about "dyspepsia and failure to thrive." There was no antibiotic treatment available until the introduction of streptomycin after 1944. In Newcastle the disease was rare in children after 1963.[6]

Dr F. J.W. Miller took a special interest in the condition with the encouragement and support of J.C. He became a leading expert and the author of many publications, including two widely distributed monographs on tuberculosis in children; one, shared with colleagues, relating to his extensive experience in Newcastle in particular between 1935 and 1970[34b] and the other from his work in South East Asia from 1966 to1979[34c]. He was a Consultant to the World Health Organisation.

Radiology

This was of vital importance in the assessment of these children, as well as other clinical problems. This was one service that J.C. failed to develop at the Babies Hospital. He lobbied hard in 1925 for the supply of an X-ray apparatus, but this was unsuccessful as there was no suitable accommodation available at the hospital. Arrangements were then made with a local company to X-ray children at 15 shillings a time, which was a relatively large fee. In 1928, on the recommendation of J.C., Dr S. Whately Davidson was appointed Honorary Radiologist. In the beginning he carried out the work 'generously' in his private practice and later, as demand increased, at Newcastle General Hospital.

Research

In 1934, in response to concerns about the high prevalence of malnutrition and infections in young children in the community, which was confirmed by his experience at the Babies Hospital, J.C. investigated the health and nutrition of children in Newcastle upon Tyne between the ages of 1 and 5 years. It was done at the request of the City Health Committee and an account is available as a chapter in the 'Selection from his writings' in 'The Purpose and Practice of Medicine' (1960).[4b] He concluded that at least 36% of the children from the poor districts of Newcastle were unhealthy or unfit and as a result appeared malnourished. The high incidence of apparent malnutrition was not found in children of 'better class' families and was therefore due to preventable causes. The immediate cause of the apparent malnutrition was the physical damage

28

done by infective diseases in susceptible young children. The main factors which promote and perpetuate this physical damage were probably:

"The housing conditions which permit mass infections of young children at susceptible ages, and improper and inadequate diet, which prevents satisfactory recovery from their illnesses."

In 1938-9, a deficient diet was still a problem in Newcastle, even though the employment of fathers had increased. Two out three families interviewed spent less on food than the cost of a basic diet.[35] In 1939, low birth weight was also a potent cause of infant mortality in addition to infections[28] which featured so frequently at the Babies Hospital. Research on the clinical problems encountered at the hospital already played a prominent part.

The short-term outcome and the length of stay [Table 1 and Figure 11]

The proportion of children who were cured on discharge home settled to an average of about 65% each year. Many others were improved; in 1936 these accounted for 30.5% of the discharges. The high mortality of about 20% throughout most of this period was due in the main to the relatively large number presenting in the late stages of disease and some already 'moribund on admission'. For many that were 'incurable', admission was sought in:

"The hope that something might be attempted for their treatment."

There really was nowhere else for them to go during those years.
By 1936, the average length of stay of the inpatients had diminished from a high of 44 days in 1927 to a low of 19 that year.

Postmortems

These were done from about 1930 by Dr A.F. Bernard Shaw, later Professor of Pathology at the RVI. He carried out the work free of charge in his spare time, mostly on Sundays and late evenings.[3] This is an example of the many freely given services and contributions, as the reputation of the Babies Hospital rose under J.C.'s leadership.
The postmortem findings in 1931 give an indication of the diseases that were identified: two bronchopneumonia, nine gastroenteritis, six tuberculosis, six sepsis and its effects, four Pink Disease, three convulsions, one each of empyema, nephritis, Hirshsprung Disease, congenital heart disease, uraemia, prematurity, bronchiectasis and pneumothorax. 16 (33%) out of the 48 infants who died that year were:

"Admitted in a hopeless state of illness and died shortly afterwards."

Lady Ridley in her memoir wrote about the special arrangements that were made[3]:

"When the committee discovered that many of the mothers could not afford to let their babies die in hospital since they could take a moribund baby home for two pence in a tram whereas the cost of transporting a coffin was prohibitive, the Committee formed a rota to undertake the transport of dead babies from the hospital in their own cars. This voluntary service continued not only throughout the 'thirties' but also all through the war when the hospital was at Blagdon Hall in Northumberland and the distance involved for the parents, not only in fetching the babies but registering their deaths at Ponteland (in Northumberland) would have been a great expense to them."

Outpatients [Table 1]

Outpatient sessions were started in 1924. During 1925-6, Monday and Friday afternoons were set aside for outpatient consultations. There was no dispensing and visits were limited to referrals from general practitioners and child welfare clinics for the purpose of a specialist opinion. The majority of admissions to the wards took place following these consultations. The number of attendances increased rapidly. J.C. commented in 1928:

"This part of the work is increasing and reveals the increased interest which is taken by the public and medical profession in the health and welfare of infants."

Mothers who were unable to leave their homes whilst their children were in hospital were encouraged to attend daily for help and advice. They also received help in re-establishing breastfeeding. Simple feeding disorders were dealt with in outpatients when the home conditions were satisfactory. Some children with rickets attended for artificial sunlight treatment with a mercury vapour lamp. Between 1933 and 1936, approximately one-third of the consultations were new referrals. There were 911 in 1936. The remainder were return visits to check progress and for further advice. The demand became so great that the number of sessions was increased to four days a week and more rooms were made available.

The outpatient notes and exchange of letters between a general practitioner and J.C. about a baby in 1939 give some indication of the nature of the consultation and the action taken by J.C. in response to a "very grave prognosis" [Figures 12a and b]. The baby turned out to have congenital syphilis. She was not admitted to hospital even though she appeared to be critically ill and sadly died at home the following day.

J.C. had advised that the baby would fare just as well at home with continued breastfeeding, which was her only chance of survival, and an oral antibiotic. Moribund babies were admitted at times, albeit with some reluctance, because of the ever present shortage of accommodation. J.C., as was his practice, took a pragmatic approach. His notes and letters are brief and to the point, as was his custom according to his contemporaries.

The family came from Durham district. That year the largest proportion of inpatients came from that district - 93 (30%) out of 307, compared with 73 (23%) from Newcastle and 69 (22%) from Northumberland. It seems that the mother had already lost a baby at the age of 6 hours and had a further child living at home. She was only 20 years old and had a positive Wasserman test (suggestive of past infection with syphilis) identified nine days after the current baby's death. It is interesting to note that the referring doctor had hinted at the diagnosis of syphilis by suggesting that she may have 'pemphigus'; a 'syphiliticus' variety was known to occur in newborn babies associated with mucocutaneous vesicles. J.C. recommended the most up to date treatment available, consisting of M and B 693, a first generation oral sulphonamide (sulphapyridine) made by May and Baker. Penicillin, which would have been the preferred bactericidal antibiotic was not available for another 4 years.

From the outset, referrals for admission came from Northumberland, Durham district, other northern districts and further afield as well as Newcastle [Figure 13 and Table 3a]. Between 1932 and 1939, the majority (between 53 and 66%) came from outside Newcastle. Private patients were also admitted unaccompanied or with their mothers or nannies. They consisted of only 2% to 7% of the referrals between 1932 and 1935, when this information was recorded (Table 3a). Fees were 'according to circumstances." There is no information about the social class of the families, nor any record of children from ethnic minorities. There were no restrictions financially or for any other reason.

As the hospital's reputation grew, there were visitors from the United Kingdom including a team from Great Ormond Street Hospital led by Dr (later Sir) Wilfred Sheldon and overseas from as far afield as the USA, New Zealand, Tokyo, Sweden and other parts of Europe. They came to see the special arrangements for the inpatient care of the babies and infants. Some were particularly interested in the pioneering surgery on cleft palate.

Visitors were made aware of the extent of infections as a potent cause of illness in infancy and the special needs of inpatient treatment when necessary. This was not universally the case in the 1920s. One hospital doctor from Manchester commented that "The Sister would be very sorry for herself if she had any of those on the ward."[3]

In 1932, three sisters from the hospital were appointed to some of the most prestigious hospitals in the country: Great Ormond Street Hospital, the Municipal Hospital for Babies in Birmingham and Vincent Square Hospital in London. The success of the service was very much due to J.C.'s leadership and he was making many contacts with colleagues and hospitals nationwide and overseas.

Education

From the beginning in 1926, education was promoted as one of the principal objectives of the Babies Hospital [Figure 15]. Medical students began to attend outpatient clinics that year and postgraduate classes were held.

J.C. and matron gave lectures open to all for a small fee. In 1927, the hospital was recognised as a teaching centre. Postgraduate classes of the Northumbria and Durham Committee were held under the scheme of the Durham Medical School. In 1929, a reciprocal arrangement was made with the Northern County School of Domestic Economy. Their housekeeping students

31

had practical experience at the hospital and nurses attended lectures in their School of Cookery. Over the years, medical students and doctors were made welcome in outpatients and ward rounds. In 1932, 38 general practitioners from Durham, Northumberland and Yorkshire and some medical students attended. The welcome to students and postgraduates in the early part of the 20th century is of historic significance. Teaching in paediatrics in Newcastle, as in most other English medical schools, did not begin until 1913 and students received only a few formal classroom lectures in the diseases of children.[18]

Between 1925 and 1939, postgraduate courses were set up by J.C. at the Babies Hospital. They were eagerly attended. It was only after the University Department of Child Health was founded in 1942 with J.C. as the first full-time Professor of Child Health in the country, that a more comprehensive course was made available.

The involvement with public bodies

Following J.C.'s first visit to the Ministry of Health in London in 1924, there were frequent contacts with this department. The ministry's approval was sought for every proposal for the development of the buildings, the acquisition of equipment and changes in the clinical service. Inspectors visited frequently. From the outset in 1926, the Ministry gave financial support as did Newcastle City Council and gradually an increasing number of the northern districts, which sent children for inpatient treatment. A municipal counsellor from Newcastle was invited to join the Committee of Management in 1931. The balance of all the yearly expenditure came from voluntary donations, fees from mothers and private patients, probationers and miscellaneous sales and fund raising events.

J.C. took an active part in the decisions about the management of the hospital. It is the reputation of the hospital, led and promoted by him, that brought such a great deal of support from local authorities, the Ministry of Health and the public. He himself sometimes contributed to the finances. The relationship with the City Health Department was further strengthened by the appointment in 1936 of Dr G. Brewis of the Newcastle Child Welfare Department, as one of the honorary assistant physicians.

The management and the finances of the hospital

The proceedings of the lay committee and detailed financial information are recorded alongside the medical and surgical reports in every Annual Report.

From the outset, women played a leading part in the management of the hospital. This was in contrast to other children's hospitals in Britain, dating from Victorian times, when women were generally not expected to assume authority and executive powers whatever their social status:

"In paediatric hospitals, they would instead often exert a powerful influence indirectly as members of ladies' committees, who visited hospitals, talked to patients and nurses, took stock of complaints, general morale, and the state of the wards. They then communicated their opinions to the hospital secretary on the board of management."[36]

The list of members of the Management Committee and the vice-presidents published in the first Annual Report of the Babies Hospital and Mothercraft Centre (1April 1925 to 31 March 1926) sets the scene for the remainder of the life of the hospital over the next 20 years:

President – The Duchess of Northumberland
Vice-presidents – 28 including 13 titled ladies, 12 lay women, one female doctor, one reverend gentleman and one male doctor
The committee – 11 lay women. The chairperson from 1929 to 1945 was Lady Ridley
J.C. as chairman of the Medical Staff Committee
The honorary secretary – Miss Greta Rowell

The honorary auditors, solicitors, bankers and treasurer were all men. J.C. encouraged and supported women during an era when men generally continued to hold the executive positions and authority in hospitals. In an unpublished memoir, Dr Errington Ellis, who had been his registrar and first assistant, recorded that J.C. had personally recommended several women, including Lady Ridley, for membership of the Committee of Management.[8]
Lady Ridley in her memoir about the Babies Hospital[3] wrote in glowing terms about the amicable collaboration with J.C. and all the members of the Hospital Management Committee. The matron, Miss Cummings, also commented:

"He was always ready to listen, nothing was too trivial for him to take notice of. He never put you off and said he hadn't time. He was a marvelous man to work for, he got the very best out of all the staff."[1]

Dr Miller also described "the courtesy, care and consideration he gave to each one of his patients" during his outpatient consultations.[5]

The receipts and payments for the year ending 31 March 1926 are shown in Figure 16. The Ministry of Health and the Newcastle Corporation provided about a third of the receipts. In addition, there were 182 individual donations that year also accounting for just over a third of the receipts. Most of these came from 162 private individuals who gave modest amounts. They included eight titled ladies, one Lord and one Knight of the Realm. There were also contributions from local businesses, welfare centres, mothers unions, schools and proceeds from charitable fundraising. The largest donation of £100 came from "A Mother." The fees paid by mothers contributed 11% to the receipts and probationers about 1%.
The sums involved increased over the years. Details of the finances during the life of the Babies Hospital from 1926 to 1945 are summarised in Appendix 3. It is noteworthy that already well before the advent of the National

Health Service in 1948, public funds contributed significantly to the finances of the hospital. During 1926 to 1930, the Ministry of Health grants accounted for about a third of the income. Thereafter, Newcastle City Council and the northern districts contributed 43% during the 1930s, rising to 57% during the war years in 1940-1944.

Despite the hardships of the Second World War, funding from local authorities increased and public donations and subscriptions continued at a high level of about 30% of the annual receipts – a tribute to the diligent work of the Committee of Management of the Babies Hospital under the chairmanship of Lady Ursula Ridley and the continuing reputation of the clinical service under the leadership of J.C. It was already recorded in the Annual Report of 1931-1932 (Appendix 2), that:

"The Hospital has the approval of the Ministry of Health," and that "In the development of the Hospital the desire of the Committee is to work in the closest cooperation with existing Health services and other institutions in the district."

Private practice was limited. The earnings of most working families were too low to sustain the expenses of inpatient treatment. Information about the proportion of private patents is limited [Table 3a]. Early in 1926-7, the proportion was 16%; during 1932-5, it was about 5% (range 1.9% to 7.5%). Mothers contributed about 7% of the income before the Second World War and then only 4% between 1940 and 1944. The approximate doubling of their contributions from 3.8% during 1928-1930 to 7.4% in 1931-1939 is accounted for by the opening of three wards for private patients in 1932. "The fees charged were according to the circumstances of the patients." There is no information about the fees paid separately to doctors.

The income often failed to match the expenditure despite great efforts at fund raising and numerous donations and subscriptions as illustrated in Appendix 3. The hospital had a persistent overdraft, readily granted by the bank. It was not cleared until the final year in 1945 with a legacy of 3000 pounds and some residual reserves.

Fundraising was difficult during the Second World War and special appeals were successfully made to increase income. The prime concerns were always the comfort of patients and staff, the acquisition and maintenance of technical equipment and the fabric of the buildings, the facilities of the hospital and the pursuit of excellence in the care of the children and their mothers. In 1932 when the overdraft was particularly high at £356 2s 7d (13.9% of the receipts), it is already recorded in the Annual Report:

"When the extra provision of the comfort of the patients and staff is taken into consideration, the Committee feel that the expenditure is justified."

It may be asserted that the successful acquisition of the funds that were required for the development and function of the Babies Hospital were, to a great extent, the direct result of the inspirational leadership of J.C. who, from the outset, promoted friendly collaboration with public institutions, the medical profession and the public at large. He thereby upheld the reputation of the hospital as a 'centre of excellence' for the care of the children and mothers of Newcastle and the northern districts.

Plans for the future

The buildings and the facilities of the hospital were always inadequate to meet the increasing demands for outpatient as well as inpatient care. After all, there was just an amalgam of adjacent terrace houses that had to be adapted for the purpose.

J.C. took the lead in the planning of a purpose-built Babies Hospital. In 1934, during a visit, an inspector of the Ministry of Health:

"Spoke in glowing terms of the work being done and encouraged the Committee to extend the premises, but strongly advised that the individuality of the Hospital be preserved."

J.C. reiterated:

"Their experience has led them to the conclusion that the arrangement, staffing, and equipment of a Babies Hospital differs entirely from that required in hospitals for older children and adults."

His intention was to plan for the accommodation for mothers in all the circumstances that required inpatient care. He expressed the hope:

"It will result in a Hospital which will serve as a model to other Hospitals in the country."

Two years later, the medical and surgical staff were collaborating with the architect in the preparation of plans for a new hospital, "which is shortly to be built." In 1937, the rebuilding scheme had been approved by the local health authorities. It was to be on or near the site of the Royal Victoria Infirmary and they were awaiting the result of an application for a grant from the Commissioner for the Special Areas.

In the event, the new hospital was never built during his lifetime. Amongst other considerations, the Second World War intervened.

An indication of what J.C. had in mind may be deduced from the plans of the new Children's Department that was opened at the nearby Newcastle General Hospital in 1938. He was appointed a consultant physician to the hospital that year and had already been involved in the initiation of the planning process. In a history of the NGH (1870-1966),[37] there is a description of the new department:

"This consists of a main block with three floors accommodating ninety-two beds, and two separate single storied wards, the quarantine ward of sixteen beds, with glass partitions dividing the ward into single-bedded cubicles, and the infants' ward with twenty beds. In this the beds are arranged both in cubicles and small wards. The axis of all the wards runs east and west and opens into the main hospital corridor. The buildings are of brick with artificial stone dressings. The wards have large glass doors giving access to commodious terraces and balconies. The main block has a number of wards that are suitable for the admission of a mother with her child, a plan that was started by Sir James Spence. The whole department was extremely well equipped and furnished."

J.C. had always taken a keen interest in the physical surroundings and facilities of children's hospitals. In his famous Charles West Lecture on 'The Care of Children in Hospitals' delivered at the Royal College of Physicians, London in 1946,[27] he concluded:

"Some members of the profession, themselves experienced in the work of children's hospitals, must make themselves expert in the physical examination of institutions. No amount of administrative or clinical experience alone will fit them for this work."

By the end of the first 12 years of the Babies Hospital, the principal clinical activities were related to the diagnosis and treatment of the wasting disorders that affected the youngest children in the community. Marasmus was one of the original conditions that prompted the start of the service. They required the most skilled nursing care and dedicated medical and surgical attention in an appropriate physical environment, which was not then available in the paediatric wards of the main hospitals in the city. In an era of still limited knowledge about the diseases of babies and infants, it took some time for specific diagnoses of organic disease to be recognised and treated. The Babies Hospital filled a yawning gap in the care of children under the age of 3 years in Newcastle and the northern districts. Older children and some younger ones were treated on the paediatric wards of the Royal Victoria Infirmary, Newcastle General Hospital and the Fleming Memorial Hospital for Sick Children. Children with fevers, such as scarlet fever and diphtheria were treated in a fever hospital at Walkergate in Newcastle.

THE BABIES HOSPITAL AT 33 WEST PARADE
IN NEWCASTLE UPON TYNE 1937 – 1939 AND AT BLAGDON HALL
IN NORTHUMBERLAND 1939 - 1945

The title of the hospital was changed in 1937 with the omission of the words 'and the Mothercraft Centre'. This was agreed by the Committee of Management in order "to avoid confusion." It did not indicate any change in policy. The age distribution amongst the inpatients remained essentially unchanged [Table 4]. 'Mothercraft' was still taught in outpatients and to the resident mothers.

The proportion of resident mothers had been increasing and by 1944 seventy mothers came in, representing 38% of new admissions. This compares with 9% ten years earlier in 1934. Feeding difficulties first recorded separately in 1933 are still recorded, albeit in decreasing numbers. The benefits of admitting mothers were again extolled by J.C., who reported that the length of stay in hospital was thereby likely to be shortened. Apart from one year in 1942 when it was three weeks, the length of stay was of the order of about two weeks [Table 4]. In the Annual Report of the Babies Hospital for 1943, J.C. wrote the most eloquent and dispassionate evaluation yet of the practice:

"The system of admitting mothers to carry out the nursing of their own infants has been continued and extended, and its value is now more than ever established. It is not too much to say that in some illnesses the lives of the children have been saved by this method of nursing by which mothers undertake the detailed care, feeding and nursing of their children under the supervision of the nursing staff. Another aspect of its value is the sense of confidence and achievement which comes to the mothers from this experience. While in Hospital each mother shares a single room with her child and the mother-child relationship remains unbroken. They leave hospital with a knowledge and experience which serves them well in after years. It is now some fifteen years since we started this system of nursing and more than a thousand mothers have shared it. As this knowledge of motherhood is handed on from family to family in the villages and towns it is difficult to overestimate its effects in family life in the North East. Nor is the value all on the side of the mothers and patients. The comradeship between mothers and professional nurses has done a great deal to establish a new outlook in the practice and technique of nursing."

Similar arrangements were also proposed after 1938 for the children's wards of the other principal hospitals in Newcastle at the Newcastle General Hospital, the Fleming Memorial Hospital for Sick Children and the Royal Victoria Infirmary. J.C. held identical views about the care of newborn babies in maternity hospitals. On his honorary appointment in 1942 to one of the city maternity hospitals, the Princess Mary Maternity Hospital, J.C. insisted that healthy mature newborn babies should no longer be routinely separated into adjacent rooms from their mothers after delivery. Their cots should remain at the bedside[38] [Figure 17]. He was "mystified by an arrangement under which their babies were away from them, when at the end of nine months waiting, they had expected to possess them."[1]

[Figure 18] illustrates the changes in the number of the individual diagnoses that were recorded amongst the children admitted to the hospital. Tables 6 to 9 provide the details. The numbers are relatively small but accurately reflect the great increase in the variety and complexity of the diagnoses that were being made. The 'miscellaneous' group constitutes only about 5% of the total. During the first two years (1937-1939), infections and infants for operation on pyloric stenosis, hare lip and cleft palate feature prominently as in previous years.

J.C. comments in 1943 on the high death rate and disablement amongst infants with serious infections such as septicaemia, gastro-enteritis and tuberculosis, which still contribute to the high infant mortality in the Tyneside area. In 1940, it was still about 65 per thousand in Newcastle compared with about 50 in England and Wales [Figure 1]. He goes on to record:

"While recognising the great saving of life and improvements in child health which have been effected in the past twenty years, it must remain a matter of concern that there should still be so much fatal and disabling disease amongst infants, diseases which might be prevented by better hygiene and care of the infants and by a wider recognition of the diseases from which they are liable to suffer."

From the outset in 1926, the lack of a complete 'cure' in the infants discharged from the hospital points to the dangers of the illnesses that afflicted them [Tables 1, 4 and Figure 11]. Up to 26% amongst the total of 1620 admitted during the six years from 1938 to 1943 were no better on discharge home or transfer to other hospitals, despite the best available treatment and care. There were many children amongst them with infections including tuberculosis at a time when sulphonamides were not generally available until after 1936, penicillin after 1943 and streptomycin after 1944.

Building on the experiences at the Babies Hospital and a survey of deaths in infancy in 1939,[28] J.C. with Dr F.J.W Miller and Dr D.C. Court and other colleagues eventually undertook a study of all the children born in May and June in 1947 in Newcastle upon Tyne.[18] The primary purpose was "to measure the frequency and extent of disease and disablement, with a view to a better understanding of the types and incidence of illness from infective causes and the conditions under which they occurred." They found that only about one-fifth of the infants escaped illness and that 86% of illnesses were infective in origin. Four conditions including respiratory infections, infective diarrhoea, skin sepsis and infectious fevers were responsible for most infections. The first two figure most prominently amongst the Babies Hospital inpatients.

In 1947, it was estimated that a quarter to a third of the work of general practitioners was concerned with sick children, mainly with respiratory infections; only 2% - 3% were referred to hospital. J.C. and his colleagues conceded that that they had little accurate knowledge of the variety and extent of illness in children in the community. It was also the intention to include "descriptions of the families, their homes and other circumstances in which they lived", in order to understand the environmental and social context in which these infections occurred. Information was therefore sought about housing, family structure, maternal capacity, infant feeding, prematurity, illegitimacy and the medical care of children in their homes, child welfare clinics and hospitals.

The original intention was to continue the study to the age of 7 years and extend the range of illnesses and disabilities to be studied. It was so successful that it carried on and continues to this day.

There was also a prime objective to record the manner in which the medical provisions for sick and healthy children were used and especially whether they met the needs of the families. The experience was to be made available for clinical teaching. It was also the intention to take the opportunity of "adjusting the invaluable experiences of health visitors or child-health nurses to the work of family doctors." It is thus evident that the 1000 Families Study contains the seeds of J.C.'s legacy as regards his contribution to the emergence of Social/Community Paediatrics as a new branch of medicine.

The main conclusion during the first stages of the Study, on the basis of a univariate analysis, was that the best correlation with health was the mother's coping ability. A more sophisticated analysis of the data, which became available later, came to a different conclusion in 1999. It was "that the rating of maternal capacity appears to have been as much a measure of the adversity experienced by the mother as of her ability to cope. Even the most satisfactory mother could do little to mitigate the insidious effects of grinding poverty."[46b]

The children continued to be followed thereafter into adulthood. Two further studies were published about their childhood up to the age of 15 years,[39] and [40] one at 32-33 years relating to the 'cycle of deprivation[41] and numerous specific studies of outcome in those who had reached the age of 50 and 60 years.[42-46]

The principal findings in adult life are that, although conditions during the antenatal period and childhood such as quality of maternal care, breast feeding, nutrition, infections and socioeconomic conditions played a part in outcomes, by the middle years of life, socio-economic factors and particularly life styles were the overwhelming determinants of physical and mental health in that population born in Newcastle in1947. Lifecourse influences differed between men and women with men at a significant disadvantage. The inclusion of aspects of lifestyle during adult life in addition to the familiar socio-economic parameters such as social class and housing are shown to be potent predictors of outcome.[44, 45] They provide a strong confirmation of the public health interventions that may contribute most to a healthy and more fulfilling life. For example, it is noteworthy that by the age of 50 years about 600 (72%) of the 832 adults, who were traced, had taken up smoking and over 50% were classified as obese. In addition to these well-established risk factors, alcohol consumption was excessive: it was estimated that 18 million units of alcohol had been consumed.[46]

The surgical operations recorded in the Annual Reports are shown in Table 9. The information is incomplete but probably represents the general trend. Very few other than infants with pyloric stenosis, hare lip and cleft palate had operations. The number of children for operation remained at the highest level of all admissions. Their mothers were admitted if at all possible. Between 1936 and 1944, the mortality of 4.4% amongst the 226 operated on for pyloric stenosis and 1.5% amongst 261 infants with hare lip and cleft palate is relatively low for that era, particularly bearing in mind the poor pre-operative condition and wasting of many of the infants.

Mr Wardill's comments on the excellent operative results bear witness to the effective and close collaboration between the medical and surgical staff, the expertise of the anaesthetists and the dedicated skill of the nursing staff:

"I grudgingly admit that without this help, the results would have made a different show. This applies equally to the Matron and her nursing staff who have always given of their best in the service of the patients."

From 1939 to 1944, the number of infants with infections is reduced. Compared with the previous decade, the number of specific diagnoses of organic disease had increased. This is a reflection of increasing knowledge and better facilities for investigation. Tuberculosis, however remained a problem.

There was also a small number of infants with 'malnutrition'. During 1940 to 1944, there were 28 and five remained for convalescence in 1945. J.C. reported in 1938 that there had been a remarkable decline in the serious forms of the condition during recent years. Rickets, which in earlier times affected the majority of the children in the poorest parts of Newcastle was by then rarely seen and the number of inpatients with this condition was very small. J.C. goes on to note:

"The improvement is due to various factors, but the most important is the research of the Medical Research Council and the clinical workers in hospital who have demonstrated clearly the methods by which the disease may be prevented."

He goes on to comment:

"While this trend of events indicates a great improvement in the nutritional state of children, it has not been accompanied by the corresponding decline in infant mortality which might have been expected. This suggests that there are factors other than malnutrition, which are responsible for the prevalent diseases and deaths among young children. This is a conclusion which is fully confirmed by our clinical studies in the Hospital in recent years."

The infant mortality rate from about 1910 to the early 1970s is shown in Figure 1. The rate in Newcastle was consistently higher than in England and Wales. During the 1920s and 1930s in particular, it rose to higher levels. This was associated with the exceptionally severe economic deprivation in the city and northern districts during that era.

40

Feeding difficulties and breastfeeding

Infants with these problems were still being admitted, albeit in decreasing numbers. J.C. was always intent on promoting breastfeeding and in 1938 published an article on 'The Modern Decline of Breast-feeding'.[47] He concluded that the decline was due to increasing indifference and mismanagement of the mother in the early stages of lactation. He went on to state:

"The correction of the fault lies mainly in the hands of those who tend and advise the mother in and shortly after her lying in. Big hospital wards and crowded child welfare clinics do not provide an atmosphere which encourages breast-feeding. Better training of doctors and maternity nurses in the care of infants may help to correct the fault; and that the importance of this education is not sufficiently recognised is suggested by the recent authoritative order of the Ministry of Health that panel practitioners attending their refresher postgraduate courses are not to receive instruction in diseases of infancy and childhood."

Nervous Diseases

The admission of children with these conditions marks a new departure for the Babies Hospital. It indicates that the clinical work was expanding into areas of more chronic yet debilitating conditions. In 1939, there were two children with 'mongolism' and one each with 'mental deficiency', hydrocephalus and convulsions. Pink Disease was included in this category. The following year in 1940, there were five children with a diagnosis of 'functional disorders' and in 1943 four with 'behaviour problems'. These are the first indications that some attention was being given at the hospital to developmental and psychological problems; a category of conditions that was to become a prominent component of later admissions to the successors of the Babies Hospital.

The transfer of the Babies Hospital to Blagdon Hall at the outbreak of the Second World War

The inpatient wards of the hospital at West Parade in Newcastle were transferred to Blagdon Hall in Northumberland in September 1939 [Figure 19]. There was imminent danger of air raids onto the nearby Vickers Armstrong munitions factories in the west of the city. A small number of cots were retained for a while at West Parade for emergency cases that could not be safely transferred.

The Hall belonged to the Ridley family and a large nursery built in 1830, as well as a kitchen area, were converted into wards. The total number of new admissions decreased by about one-third during the war, but the number of operations for pyloric stenosis, hare lip and cleft palate as well as the number of children with tuberculosis and rickets remained at about the same level. An Honorary Assistant Surgeon, Mr Cowell, had been appointed in 1938. He was 'on active service' during the war, leaving Mr Wardill to undertake the surgery.

The largest decrease was in the number of infections, which diminished by about 70%, with respiratory tract infections, gastroenteritis and dysentery

41

significantly less prominent. The proportion of children in the different age groups, including the youngest under the age of 4 months, remained unchanged. The decrease in the number of infections was most likely due to the admission of more of these acutely ill children who were resident in Newcastle to the city's hospitals in preference to 7 miles away at Blagdon Hall. The sharp drop in the total number of admissions of Newcastle residents to the Babies Hospital during this time is in keeping with this view.

Temporary partitions were installed to maintain the principle of giving individual nursing care in a separate room to each baby and infant, accompanied by the mother whenever possible. As in the couple of years before the war, about a third of the children came to stay with their mothers, notwithstanding the change of location to a less accessible hospital in rural Northumberland [Table 4]. In 1942, the verandah from the Babies Hospital in Newcastle was dismantled and re-erected at the Hall. It continued to accommodate up to six cots, which were set aside for long-stay tuberculous infants and the few with severe rickets. Children were now able to sleep out in the summer and the routine was organised exactly as a healthy children's nursery. It is recorded:

"The improvement in the children's general and psychological health under these conditions has been most remarkable."

The extensive gardens and grounds were used to advantage [Figure 20]. The huts in the garden enabled some of the children to be out all day during the summer months.

The conduct of research was most affected by the war. Nevertheless, J.C. still took the opportunity in the new surroundings at Blagdon Hall to increase knowledge and expertise. In 1943, he wrote:

"In spite of the war and its restrictions we have been able to advance still further our arrangements for dealing with the patients who because of the nature of their illnesses have to stay for long periods in Hospital. Most of these are children from tuberculous households for whom we have to make this provision. Special wards and nursing arrangements are set aside to deal with this problem. We have learnt a great deal from this. No longer is it sufficient merely to provide adequate wards, verandahs and balcony sleeping quarters. To this must be added opportunities for daily excursions whether in prams or by walking. This is not a matter of sentiment but a logical step towards better nursing arrangements. We have been fortunate that the war has placed the hospital in a house and environment in which we had the opportunity to make these trials and advances."

In 1945, as Blagdon Hall was used exclusively for patients requiring convalescent care and nursing over a long period, J.C. used the temporary hospital for a study of age grouping of children under nursery conditions [Figure 21].

During the war, the honorary medical and surgical staff had to man the hospital without the assistance of a resident doctor until 1944, when Dr Mary Taylor, was appointed. There had been a resident medical officer at the hospital in Newcastle since 1927 and all the consultants, including J.C., did a ward round of the whole hospital on the day of their outpatient clinics.[3] Two of the incumbents, Dr Elsie Wright and Dr A.G. Ogilvie were later appointed Honorary Assistant Physicians. Dr Taylor visited the hospital at Blagdon almost every day until her residence. A weekly rota of the consultant staff was organised for emergencies day and night and fortnightly for the routine work. The round trip of 14 miles from Newcastle was sometimes a problem, but the clinical work and the surgery were not significantly affected.

The honorary medical and surgical staff

From the outset, J.C. attracted physicians and surgeons to work at the hospital, who became some of the leading consultants in Newcastle in later years [Table 24]. The insights that they gained about the care of children in hospital spread further afield.

The sources of referral, 1939 to 1944 [Tables 3a and b, and Figure 13]

During the years of the Second World War and the transfer to Blagdon Hall in Northumberland, there was a decrease in the total number of admissions and in the proportion of admissions from Newcastle. There had been a progressive decline in the admissions of Newcastle residents from 44% during 1926 -1935, to 30% during 1936 - 1939, and down to 18% in 1940 -1944.[11] It is likely that the sharp decrease in the number of admissions during the war, especially of Newcastle residents, was due in part to the practical difficulties associated with the distance and difficulties of access for some mothers living in the city. Facilities for babies and infants and accommodation for mothers in Newcastle had also increased, especially after the opening of the purpose built Children's Department at Newcastle General Hospital in 1938 and the appointment there of J.C. as consultant physician. That year too, Dr George Davison was the paediatric registrar there; he was one of the honorary assistant physicians at the Babies Hospital from 1940 and later consultant at NGH after 1947. A fifth of the admissions came from Northumberland and a handful from as far afield as Yorkshire, Cumberland, Hampshire, Derby and Scotland. The reputation of J.C and that of the hospital was now well established.

In August 1944, a disastrous fire occurred at Blagdon Hall. The wards were not affected, but all the children had to be transferred to the children's wards in Newcastle (the NGH and RVI) and the wartime Emergency Medical Service Hospital at Lancaster. J.C. led the emergency arrangements and helped to fight the fire.

In the meantime outpatients continued to be seen in Newcastle at West Parade until July 1943, when the service transferred to the Children's Clinic at the RVI. Clinical observations were still proceeding. In 1940, J.C. reported:

43

"The Outpatient Department and its work has not been affected by the war. It has continued as a consultative centre for patients sent by their family doctors or by the Medical Officers of Welfare Centres. The number of attendances has not fallen below the pre-war level and includes a number of women and babies who have sought refuge in the district from heavily bombed towns in other parts of the country. From the work of the Outpatient Department a fairly accurate impression can be gained of the prevalence of sickness and disease amongst young children in the district. Our experiences in the past year has shown that up to the present, the war has produced no ill-effects on the health of the children. There has been no evidence of disease due to inadequate diet or the restrictions of rationing."

A few months after the fire, a ward was re-opened at Blagdon Hall for long-stay convalescent cases, including infants with tuberculosis and chronic respiratory tract infections [Table 6]. These hospital facilities finally closed in the middle of 1946.

Nutrition

The clinical work at the Babies Hospital required a thorough expertise in nutrition. J.C. left a legacy of improved knowledge and practice, which he taught to the medical profession and the public.

His first publication in 1930 on nutritional xerophthalmia and night-blindness in 17 patients included two children aged 2 years amongst the 11 under the age of 14 years.[4c] He found a significant dietary deficiency probably due to inadequate vitamin A intake, associated with insufficient animal fat and meat protein in the diet. He also found an unusual high incidence of infections amongst 99 family members over a period of two years. A high incidence of skin infections and epithelial cells in the urine were prominent clinical findings amongst those with the disease. Curative treatment consisted of cod liver oil with additional milk and butter.

Four years later, he undertook the survey of the health and nutritional status of children aged 1-5 years in Newcastle, which has already been described.[4b] Defective nutrition was still a problem in 1938-39.[35]

In July 1940, in a seminal lecture before the Royal Institution entitled 'The Nation's Larder in Wartime'[48] J.C. described the composition of foods suitable for the health and growth of children. He comments:

"The stresses and strain of war experiences are not those which interfere with breast feeding. Indeed, by a wise biological adjustment, the absence of a husband at the war seems to have the effect of bringing out more strongly a woman's maternal qualities."

He gave detailed advice on the feeding of infants, reiterating:

"At least 95% of women will be able to feed their children if they desire to do so and are not misled by their attendants."

He went on to describe optimal diets during the second year and later in childhood pointing out that in the days of rationing these provide:

"More than enough of body-building and protective foods, to carry in them a considerable factor of safety."
Commenting further:

"For many years past, through poverty and ignorance, large numbers of children in this country have lived on diets deficient in proteins and other body-building foods."

He went on to write:

"Whatever may happen in the future, it is unlikely that food supplies will be so restricted as to cause a general lowering of children's diets to these levels. But the greater the restrictions the more need there will be to measure carefully the basic requirements of each child and to distribute the available food wisely and economically."
In the event, unlike in continental Europe,[49, 50] the increasing restrictions and rationing of the war did not materially affect the nutrition and wellbeing of children in Britain.[51] Measures were taken to ensure that an adequate and appropriate diet with additional vitamins was given to children together with pregnant and nursing mothers. The essential foods were distributed as fairly as possible to the entire population in the country. J.C. made a valuable contribution with Dr F.J.W. Miller by advising the Ministry of Health on the guidelines for the implementation of the National Milk Scheme. Provision was made for the distribution of liquid milks for school children and half and full cream dried milk for bottle fed infants The milk was fortified with vitamins A and D and orange juice which contained vitamin C.[51] Problems arose when there were considerable objections to the restriction of the manufacturers' guidance solely to advice about the reconstitution of powder to cow's milk. Dr Miller describes the 'degree of skill' deployed by J.C. in order to arrive at a reasonable solution 'in a very sensitive situation."[7b] As a result of all these measures, the health and growth of children improved, the infant mortality diminished and the health and longevity of adults increased in comparison with the conditions that existed before the war.[51] J.C.'s publicity about appropriate nutrition for children was very welcome.

A clinical research department

In 1936, J.C. drew attention to the pressing need for a Department of Clinical Investigation and Research. Already 10 years earlier, he had persuaded the Management Committee to convert a garage into a laboratory. The £100 donated by 'a mother' in 1926 went towards the £250 required to complete the work. Clinical assistants to help in the routine clinical work were later appointed. He was seeking special funds of at least £1000 a year over the next few years. The funds were rapidly forthcoming and two years later in 1938, the department was opened at the Babies Hospital at West Parade. It was supported by the Medical Research Council, who sent one of their researchers, Dr Jean Cass, to work there. J.C. pointed out the need for such a development by emphasising:

"The attention which has been given to the national problem of physical fitness. It is apparent to some that a good deal of the poor physique and ill health amongst young adults is due to diseases and other causes which operate in early childhood. It is a relic of ill health in infancy. It is reasonable to ask that a very small proportion of the vast sums of money which are spent in attempting to provide physical fitness in adults should be devoted to the study of the very cause of unfitness. It is doubtful whether throughout the whole country more than a few hundred pounds are being spent each year in direct medical research into the problems of diseases in infancy. It is to correct this appalling defect that we seek to establish a department of clinical research at the Babies Hospital."

The plans for the future

In July 1938, an agreement was signed for the amalgamation of the Babies Hospital with the Royal Victoria Infirmary and the Fleming Memorial Hospital to form a joint children's hospital. At the outbreak of the war, the scheme for rebuilding was postponed. In 1939, J.C. was appointed Honorary Consultant Physician to the Infirmary. Following the fire at Blagdon Hall in 1944, there was a hope that a temporary building scheme above the children's wards of the RVI would provide accommodation for the Babies Hospital, now that it was formally amalgamated with that main hospital. This did not materialise and eventually a new Babies Hospital was opened in May 1948 close to the RVI site at Leazes Terrace. This resembled the original hospital at West Parade. Two terrace houses were joined together with an initial provision for 13 patients. Later a third adjacent house was added. The building of a combined children's hospital to include all the paediatric wards in Newcastle was now on hold. It did not come about until more than six decades later on the RVI site.

The Nuffield Chair of Child Health in Newcastle

J.C. accepted the invitation in 1942 by the School of Medicine in Newcastle upon Tyne, which was connected with Durham University, to be the first whole-time Professor of Child Health in the country. In 1963, it came to be associated with Newcastle University. His work and experience at the Babies Hospital had contributed significantly to the foundation of his reputation as a clinician, an educator, a researcher and an administrator. Dr F.J.W. Miller wrote that J.C.:

"Chose to call his new University Department the Nuffield Department of Child Health. For this title carried a declaration that its work was not to be bounded by the responsibilities of the care of sick children in hospital and the teaching of students, but would include within its purpose and survey the investigation, classification and description of the social background of illness and the conditions for healthy development."[7a]

Sir John Charles in his memoir (1960) detailed the influential national committees to which he had already been appointed. These included the Curtis Committee on Child Care, the Nuffield Provincial Hospitals Trust Medical Advisory Department Committee, the Committee on Medical Education of the Royal College of Physicians, the College's Committee on Social and Preventative Medicine, where he was chairman and the Goodenough Committee on Education. He had already done research on rickets for the Medical Research Council[33] and in 1944 was invited to be one of its clinical members. He was also a member of the Universities Grant Committee and a founding member of the British Paediatric Association in 1928.

He was now in a position to develop a comprehensive Department of Child Health in Newcastle with a unified hospital service for children. There was the prospect of promoting more widely the education of the medical profession, as well as the research into the causes, prevention and treatment of the diseases of childhood.

The contributions of J.C. to clinical practice and hospital organisation at the Babies Hospital.

In the penultimate Annual Report of 1944 of the Babies Hospital, J.C. was intent on establishing two important principles. He wrote:

"The first is the management of the clinical ward in a combined clinical unit in which paediatric physicians are responsible for the organisation of the work and the routine care of the patients, acting in close co-operation with surgeons and specialists. This arrangement has to be based on the understanding that clinical paediatrics is one of the most difficult and highly technical branches of general medicine and surgery, and requires a special training and experience for those who undertake it.

The second principle is the provision of accommodation with carefully planned single rooms to which mothers can be admitted to enable them to carry on the nursing of their own sick children. For more than fifteen years these methods have been applied in the Babies Hospital and the value and success of the methods is now beyond question."

He was concerned not just with the needs of the child, but also with the emotional needs of the mother. Two years later in 1946, in the Convocation Lecture of the National Children's Home, entitled "The Purpose of the Family",[52] he commented:

"The materials needed for emotional development are every bit as important as those for physical development."

These comments about emotional development will be referred to again later in a discussion of J.C.'s apparent lack of a proper understanding of this aspect of children's development, as suggested by a leading psychologist during the 1950s.

This lecture, which is worthy of careful study as a synopsis of his understanding of family life, points the way to the conditions necessary for optimal growth and development and the contribution of medicine to pursue that objective. His teachings at the Babies Hospital and the example that he set were an inspiration to medical students and all those who came into contact with the hospital.

One further principle may be highlighted. His understanding of the crucial importance not just of family life, but also the social-environmental influences that affect the health and welfare of children.

Amongst all the advances in clinical practice that J.C. promoted, the attention to breastfeeding and nutrition which were so successfully supervised by the nursing staff in the many wasted babies treated at the hospital, stands out as a crucial element in the success of the service.

The Babies Hospital only ever dealt with a relatively small number and proportion of the youngest children from Newcastle and the northern districts, who required admission to hospital for treatment. Some could not be admitted at times due to a shortage of accommodation. Very few, if any, were over the age of 3 years. Most were under the age of 3 months. Nonetheless, during a period of 20 years when there was still a high infant mortality and morbidity in the north eastern communities, a grand total of 4805 were admitted during 1925 to 1945. The number built up to an average of 340 per year between 1936 and 1939, but fell to 229 per year during the Second World War years at Blagdon Hall [Tables 3a and b].

During the 1920s and 1930s according to J.C., the hospital provided about half the number of cots that were then available in Newcastle and the northern districts for the inpatient treatment of children under the age of 3 years. It is evident that the hospital under his leadership was a highly sought after service and a beacon of excellence by virtue of the quality of care, the efficient organisation, the emphasis on research and education and the ethos of humane service to the children and their mothers. The latter were welcomed into residence and daily visiting was encouraged if they were unable to stay with their children.

Finally, the overwhelming impression on reading all the commentaries in the Annual Reports of the Committee of Management and those of J.C. and the surgeon Mr Wardill is of a happy, purposeful hospital, which J.C. led from the front and where all concerned worked harmoniously together for the benefit of their patients. This is one of his enduring legacies [Figure 22].

THE BABIES HOSPITAL AT LEAZES TERRACE 1948 - 1976

Two adjacent terrace houses were adapted as at the first Babies Hospital at West Parade. Mothers were accommodated [Figure 24] and were able to take their children out to Leazes Park across the road [Figures 23a and 23b]. The hospital was situated close to the Royal Victoria Infirmary. The children's outpatient department was located conveniently in the grounds of the Infirmary and this building also contained the elements of J.C.'s Child Health Department. There was accommodation there for him, his secretary and Dr Miller and Dr Court, his principal colleagues in the University department. There was also a library, which became the meeting place for all members of his department and the many visitors that came to see him.

Professor Donald Court, who succeeded him after his untimely death in 1954, took the lead. Paediatricians who had been appointed by J.C., including Dr Gerald Neligan and Dr Christine Cooper, joined him to look after children at the hospital. Outpatients continued to be seen at the Children's Clinic at the RVI.

During the first seven years at Leazes Terrace up to 1955, the number and proportion of children with infections was relatively high (about 30%) and comparable to those in the pre-war years (1933-1938) [Tables 2, 6 and 10]. As the number of admissions with infections receded, children with an increasing range of medical conditions continued to be admitted for investigation and treatment [Figure 25]. This was the result of increasing knowledge, specialisation and means of diagnosis. However in 1950, there were still seven admissions for Pink Disease in which the cause had not yet been determined. There was still a great need for the hospital treatment of babies and infants with infections. A survey of all the children under the age of 12 years admitted to Newcastle hospitals and nursing homes over a two year period in 1943-1944 had been initiated by J.C.[27] It highlighted the necessity still of significant inpatient facilities for admissions related to infections; 77% of all admissions in Newcastle [Table 11], a situation that still persisted for some years after the war. Tuberculosis in infants was still a problem until the early 1960s. Large numbers of children continued to be referred to The Children's Outpatient Clinic at the RVI [Figures 26a and b].

An increasing number of newborn babies were admitted up to the early 1960s. This included a number with Rhesus haemolytic disease before the regional service for mothers and babies for these conditions was fully established at the Princess Mary Maternity Hospital in Newcastle by Dr W. Walker (Later Professor of Haematology).[38]

Surgery which had such a prominent place at the hospital under J.C. - 38% of all admissions during 1937 to 1944 - did not resume at Leazes Terrace until the appointment of a consultant paediatric surgeon in 1960, Mr J. E. S. Scott, one of the first in the country. Before then, the few referred to the hospital, who required an operation were transferred to the NGH and RVI. By 1965, the surgical cases represented an even higher proportion (66%) of the admissions to the hospital than in earlier years [Table 10]. This was due to a new regional surgical service for newborn babies with non-cardiac conditions, older children with urinary tract problems and many common conditions such as hernias as day cases. Cardiac problems were operated on later at Freeman Hospital in Newcastle and paediatric cardiology was established there by 1973.

A second consultant paediatric surgeon, Mr J. Wagget, was appointed in 1970. The residential facilities for mothers were in great demand during those years; 70% of the children admitted in 1976 (up to November) came in with their mothers [Table 10]. From 1971, the surgical service transferred in stages to the Fleming Memorial Hospital as the facilities at the old terrace houses that made up the hospital were no longer fit for purpose. By 1973 just before the final transfer, about a third of all surgical admissions included babies and infants for major operations for tracheo-oesophageal fistula, diaphragmatic hernia and Hirshsprung disease. As at the Babies Hospital during the 1930s, expert anaesthesia was an essential component of the service. During the 1950s, Dr J. Inkster (consultant anaesthetist) developed a new technique to assist the artificial ventilation of immature babies with very small airways. By the addition of a small resistance during the baby's expiration, the lungs were prevented from fully deflating to such an extent that the lower airways remained open for longer, with significant improvement in oxygenation. After the presentation of these findings to the World Congress of Anaesthesia in 1968, "positive end expiratory pressure" (PEEP) was introduced worldwide and extended to adults.[138] He also designed with Sister Lynda Maybee a ventilator that could be dismantled for sterilisation and then readily re-assembled. This was a major factor in the prevention of infection. Plastic surgery for hare lip and cleft palate never returned to the Babies Hospital after 1944; the service was relocated to the RVI and eventually transferred to the Fleming Memorial Hospital.

The report of admissions in 1955 [Table 12] is noteworthy because it gives a detailed account of a new group of conditions, which came to the fore at the Babies Hospital. A handful of infants under the label of 'functional disorders' and 'behaviour problems' had been admitted for assessment and treatment during 1940-1944 [Table 6]. By 1950, there were 16 with management and behaviour problems [Table 10]. Amongst the eight who were 'mismanaged', there was one whose mother was ill with her infant being looked after by the 14-year-old sister and four were associated with infections. The eight with 'behaviour problems' were infants with poor sleep, constant crying and 'lack of control'. The report of 1955 was written by Dr Leonard Strang, the paediatric registrar, later to become the first professor of paediatrics in an undergraduate medical school in London at University College Hospital. There were 26 admissions with 'behaviour disorders and problems of management' that year [Table 12]. He described two case histories:

(A) "A mother had her first child in a town 50 miles away. The baby at 10 weeks became ill, jaundiced and lost weight. He was taken to hospital where he was first taken in for 2 months. Although the mother was allowed to visit daily, she was never to handle or feed her baby. The baby's jaundice faded, but he didn't gain weight, so that by 5½ months he was a tiny living skeleton of only 8½

Infant Mortality Rate

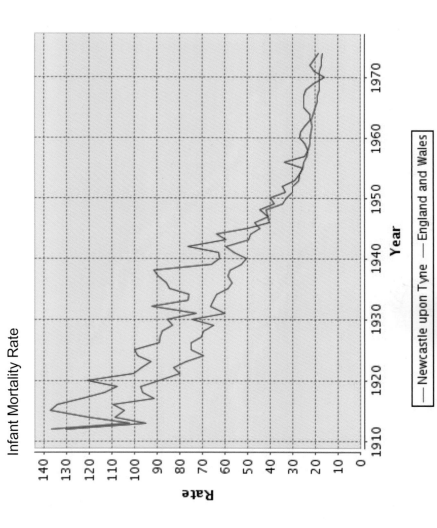

Figure 1: "A Vision of Britain through Time", c.1910-1970.
GB Historical GIS/University of Portsmouth and Newcastle upon Tyne

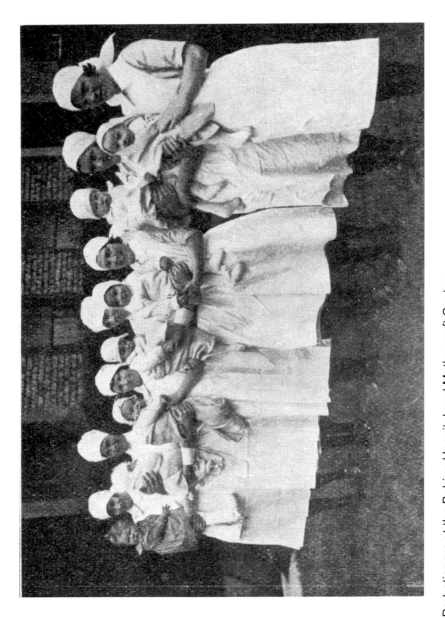

Figure 2: Probationers at the Babies Hospital and Mothercraft Centre. Annual Report. 1930-1931

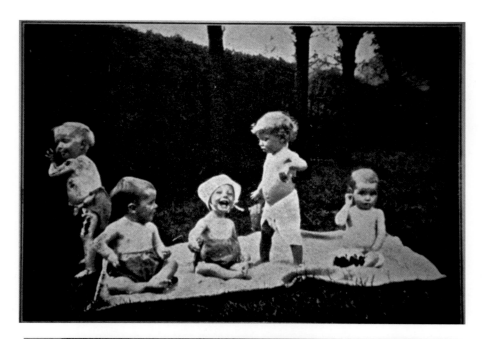

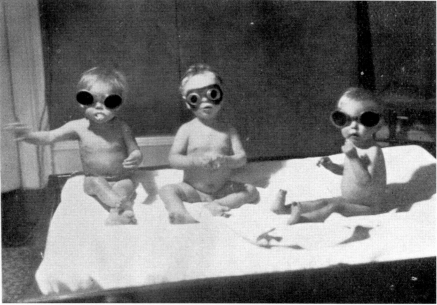

Figures 3a and 3b: The Babies Hospital and Mothercraft Centre.
Sunbathing in the garden and sunray treatment with mercury vapour lamp for rickets
Annual Report. 1927-1928

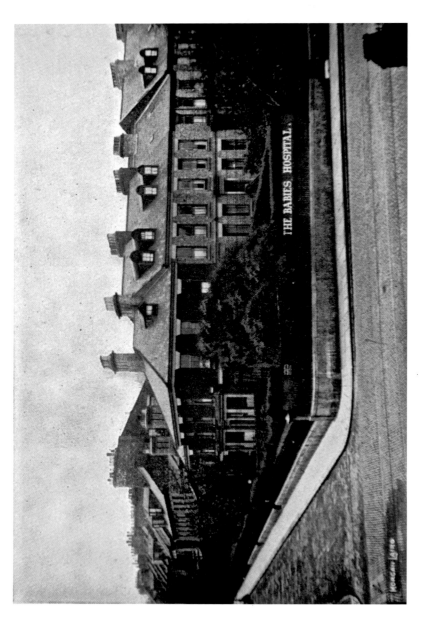

Figure 4: The Babies Hospital and Mothercraft Centre at 33 West Parade, Newcastle - upon - Tyne Annual Report. 1936 - 1937

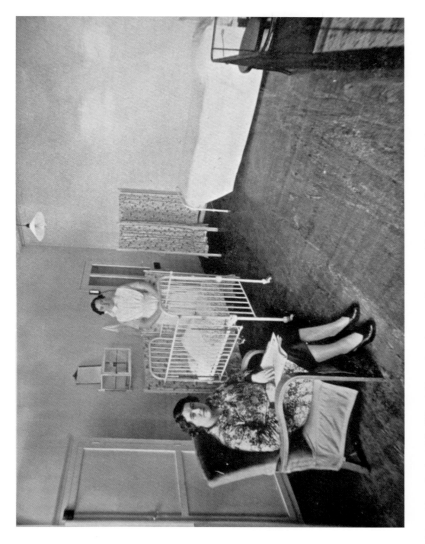

Figure 5: The Babies Hospital at 33, West Parade. A room for a resident mother and baby Annual Report 1938

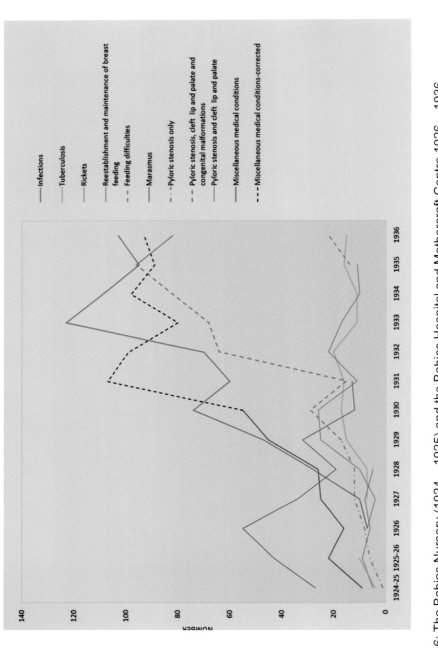

Figure 6: The Babies Nursery (1924 – 1925) and the Babies Hospital and Mothercraft Centre 1926 – 1936
The changing pattern of diagnoses

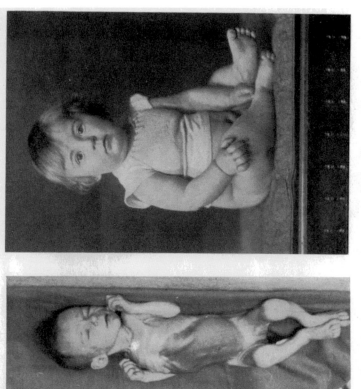

4½ lbs. at 7 weeks.

19 lbs. 13 ozs. at 1 year.

Figure 7: An example of an Infant treated in The Babies Hospital and Mothercraft Centre
Marasmus
Annual Report 1933

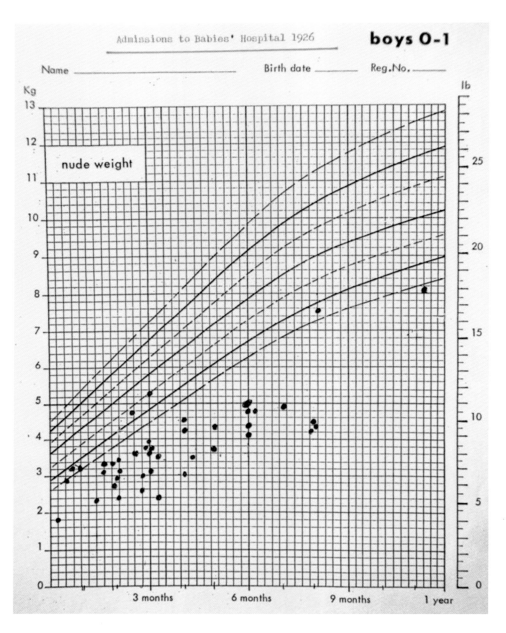

Figure 8: The weight of boys on admission from the records of the Babies Hospital and Mothercraft Centre. 1926

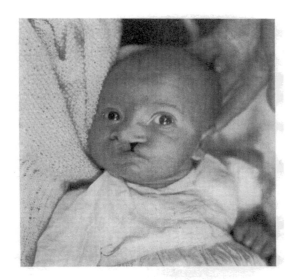

BEFORE OPERATION.

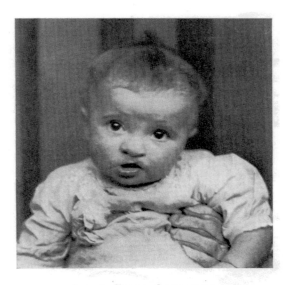

AFTER FIRST OPERATION.

Figure 9: The Babies Hospital and Mothercraft Centre
Hare lip and cleft palate
Annual Report 1933 - 1934

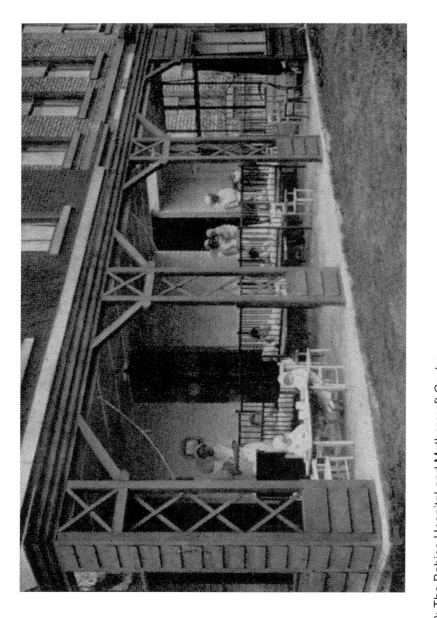

Figure 10: The Babies Hospital and Mothercraft Centre
The verandah paid for by the collection of a mile of pennies
Annual Report 1935 - 1936

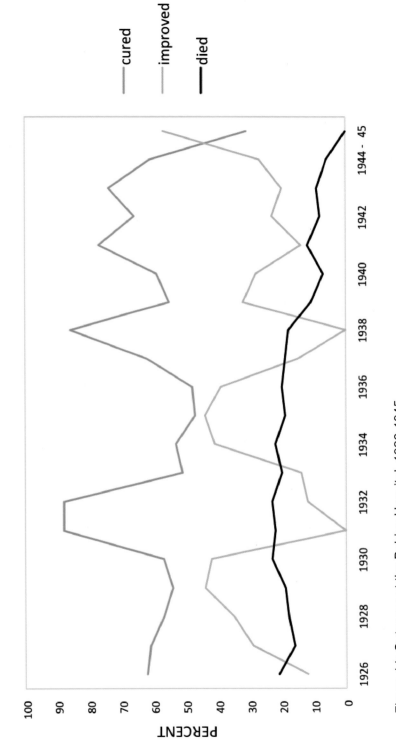

Figure 11: Outcome at the Babies Hospital. 1926-1945

THE BABIES' HOSPITAL,

NEWCASTLE-ON-TYNE.

O.P. No.	Date of Birth. _Sept 39_
7/11	Name. _Victoria_ Age. _2/52_
	Address.
Date.	
11.10.39.	Sent by _Dr McIntyre_
	Father's Employment _H. M. Forces_

DIAGNOSIS :

Cong. S.

NOTES :

M. 20: a Russian: _[illegible]_ _[illegible]_

F. 29, a soldier.

married 2 yrs ago in Pekin.

① d. @ 6 hr. a prem. Nov 1938

② 3rd ch.

Born at home, _[illegible]_ _[illegible]_ of nurse.

mothers blood Taken on 20.10.39 for W.R.

Blood W.R. is Positive. Child died at home 12.10.39.

31.10.39 - Letter to Dr McIntyre.

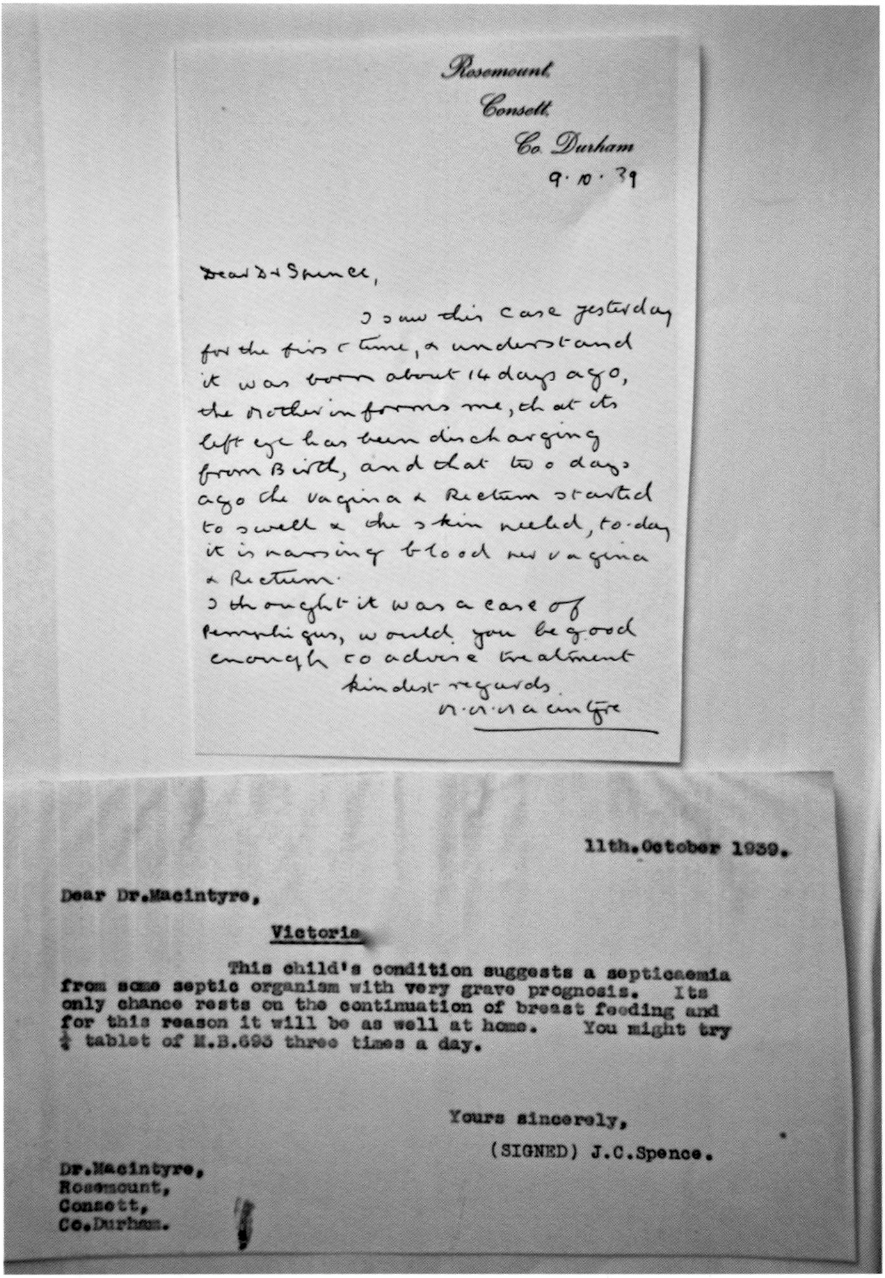

Rosemount
Consett
Co. Durham
9·10·39

Dear Dr Spence,

I saw this case yesterday for the first time, & understand it was born about 14 days ago, the mother informs me, that its left eye has been discharging from birth, and that two days ago the vagina & rectum started to swell & the skin peeled, to-day it is passing blood per vagina & rectum.
I thought it was a case of pemphigus, would you be good enough to advise treatment
kindest regards.
D. Macintyre

11th. October 1939.

Dear Dr. Macintyre,

                    Victoria

         This child's condition suggests a septicaemia from some septic organism with very grave prognosis. Its only chance rests on the continuation of breast feeding and for this reason it will be as well at home.   You might try ½ tablet of M.B.693 three times a day.

                              Yours sincerely,

                                 (SIGNED) J.C.Spence.

Dr. Macintyre,
Rosemount,
Consett,
Co. Durham.

Figure 12b: The Babies Hospital
Exchange of letters between Sir James Spence and family doctor 1939

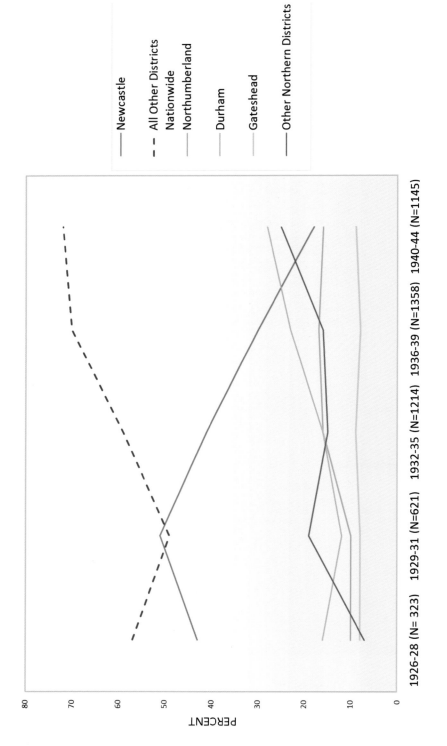

Figure 13: Sources of Referral to the Babies Hospital 1926-1944

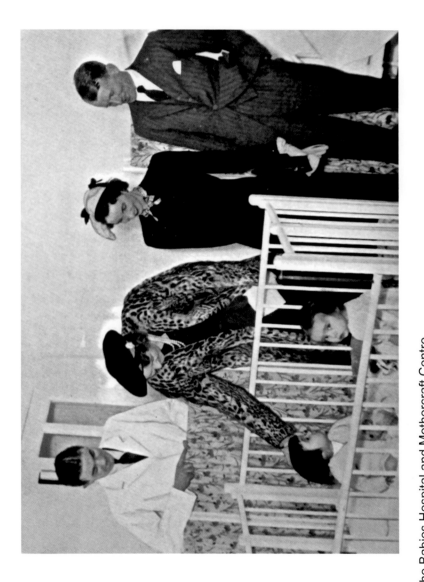

Figure 14: The Babies Hospital and Mothercraft Centre.
Visitors to the hospital. Dr G. Brewis (Honorary Assistant Physician), a visitor, Lady Ridley and Dr James Spence
Annual Report. 1937

THE BABIES' HOSPITAL and MOTHERCRAFT CENTRE.

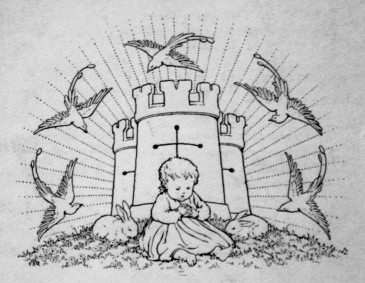

33, WEST PARADE,
NEWCASTLE-ON-TYNE.

ANNUAL REPORT,
April 1st, 1925, March 31st, 1926.

The Objects of the Hospital are :—

1.—To provide Hospital treatment for Babies suffering from diseases and disorders of nutrition.

2.—To provide opportunities for research into the means by which the prevalent diseases and mortality among infants may be prevented.

3.—To teach the principles of the care and treatment of infants.

4.—To train girls in the care of infants.

Daily Bros. & Co., Ltd., Printers, Newcastle

Figure 15: The First Annual Report 1925 - 1926

lbs. The difficulty of our colleagues at the other hospital was that no diagnosis could be found to meet the failure to thrive. When the mother came to us with her baby, we did only two things, tried our best to make a diagnosis – and in that we failed; allowed the mother the care of her own baby – the mother did not fail; within a fortnight she was able to go home with the baby gaining weight, and she has continued to gain and thrive since then."

(B) "C.D. was the 6th child – five years separated him from the nearest in the family. His mother was over 50 and harassed by the anxiety of a sick mother, a mentally unstable sister, a husband in dangerous work as a steeple-jack and a damp house in Park Road (in Newcastle). From the age of 2 weeks, the baby never settled – never slept properly, fed poorly and cried incessantly, keeping all the family awake. Nerves became frayed and tensions mounted over the months so that at 11 months, when admitted with her baby to the Babies Hospital, the mother was near distraction. By a gradual process we were able to get to know the mother and enable her to understand how tensions in the family affected her baby's behaviour. We then arranged for separation of the mother and baby for a short period, during which time she had a rest to sort out her personal and domestic life. The baby was transferred to a fairly normal atmosphere in our nursery and began to sleep well, and when he finally went home to a much calmer house, he continued in this improved habit."

This is an important milestone, as it denotes a fundamental new addition to the work of the hospital. The other children's wards in the main hospitals in the city were dealing as always with the great number of the prevalent acute infections and organic diseases in older children and in accidents. Resources and expertise in the assessment and management of behaviour disorders were limited. At the Babies Hospital, the nursing staff - as a result of the experience of their contacts with the resident mothers - had acquired an understanding of family and social circumstances, which allied to the close attention of the paediatricians were thus able to provide a sought after service.

Dr Christine Cooper. OBE, MA, BChir, Cantab, DCH, FRCP[53]

During the 1970s, there began the admission of children who had been physically abused and neglected or were at serious risk of harm at the hands of their parents or caretakers. In 1976, there is a record of 8 children who had been harmed and 12 who were receiving poor care at home. The experience of the staff and the ambience of the hospital were suited to this new development, which was initiated by Dr Christine Cooper [Figure 27]. She was the first consultant in Newcastle to take a special interest in child protection and the care of vulnerable children from dysfunctional families. She came to be recognised as the principal paediatric expert in Newcastle and the northern region.

Her career started as a nursery nurse student and she then went on to train as a doctor in London. Her connection with J.C. began in 1950 when she came to Newcastle as his senior registrar. The following year, she succeeded Dr

Elsie Wright as consultant to the Children's Department at Newcastle General Hospital. Professor Court writes:

"She was captivated by the personality of James Spence and that this determined much of her future professional thinking."[54]

During a stay in Sierra Leone during 1964 to 1966, when she was invited to advise on the development of their child health services, she gained a considerable understanding of the effects of poor environmental conditions and family deprivations. She was awarded the OBE for these services. She also realised that she needed much more knowledge and understanding of the emotional life of children and their families. She joined a group of younger paediatricians under the leadership of Anna Freud who met regularly for ten years in the latter's home in Hampstead in London and concerned themselves with the psychoanalytic aspects of children's development. In 1972, she was a member of the Houghton Committee on Adoption that recommended important changes to the law[55] and became the medical adviser to the Northern Counties Adoption Society.

She also gained invaluable experience and help through her contact with Professor Henry Kempe and his team at the University of Colorado, USA. These were pioneers in the identification and management of child abuse and neglect.[56] Physicians had been aware for several centuries of the possibility that children were at times physically abused and neglected by their parents or caretakers.[57] However, it was not until after the publication by Professor Kempe and his colleagues in 1962 of the description of the Battered Child Syndrome[58] that the medical profession took concerted action to identify the problem and protect children. During the 1960s and early 1970s in the United Kingdom, as elsewhere in the world:

"Awareness outside the medical profession was very limited and members of the legal and social welfare agencies were not involved centrally. The emphasis of social work was still to keep families together and to prevent delinquency."[59]

The National Society for the Prevention of Cruelty to Children (NSPCC), founded in Liverpool in 1883 followed by a London Society in 1885, was already dealing with referrals of suspected cases from hospitals during the later part of the nineteenth century and very large numbers from the community thereafter.

Dr Cooper was amongst the first paediatricians in Britain to recognise the nature and extent of child abuse and neglect and take practical steps to protect children and help vulnerable families.[60] She was an active member of the Tunbridge Wells Study Group convened in 1973 by Dr Alfred White Franklin (consultant paediatrician) to consider the way forward in child protection. This was an influential paediatric initiative in collaboration with the NSPPC, which had already established its own Battered Child Research Unit in 1968. It attracted the attention of the central government and Sir Keith Joseph, the Secretary of State for Social Services and senior officials of the Department of Health and

Social Security (DHSS) attended the first meeting. At the conclusion of the meeting, an inquiry into the circumstances of the tragic death of Maria Colwell (see below) was announced as well as the foundation of The British Association for the Study of Child Abuse and Neglect.[61] Dr Cooper became the president of the Association in due course.

It was well known in Newcastle that when she began her work with children who had been abused and neglected, which led to the need to give evidence in court, magistrates and their clerks regarded those who recognised the danger to children as unnaturally prejudiced. Dr Cooper spoke and lectured widely about these problems and medical students and many others were shown graphic slides of young children that she had encountered with non-accidental bruises and fractures who were later killed by their parents and caretakers. She was a prominent member of the Newcastle Social Services Committee, which developed guidelines for the identification by health, social, education and legal services of non-accidental injuries and neglect. Most of these were adopted by Social Services and the medical profession nationwide.

Her work later at the Mother and Child Unit at the Fleming Hospital from 1977 to 1983 was part of the many influential activities related to child protection in which she was involved. In 1985, following her retirement, she contributed a section entitled, 'Good enough, borderline and bad enough parenting' in a book dedicated to the subject.[62]

Before the admission of vulnerable children to the Babies Hospital at Leazes Terrace, there is only one record throughout the twenty years of the original Babies Hospital of the admission of an infant with child protection issues. In October 1927, an infant of 7 months from Byker in Newcastle was sent in by the NSPCC with diarrhoea and vomiting. She weighed 14 lb 8 oz. Fourteen days later she was "removed against medical advice." She had lost over one pound and weighed only 13 lb 6 oz. It has not been possible to obtain any further relevant data and she may not have survived.

The NSPCC, as in other parts of the country, was already very active in Newcastle and the northern region during the early years of the 20th century. The extent of this involvement is quite startling and indicates the considerable reservoir of vulnerable children at risk of abuse and neglect, which did not engage the active clinical attention of paediatric services of Newcastle and the northern region until the second half of the 20th century. On 22 August 1919, the Evening Chronicle in Newcastle published a brief report about the Society. The local information and the total numbers of referrals and adult offenders in the country are staggering.

"The National Society for the Prevention of Cruelty to Children investigated 3146 complaints of neglect and cruelty in England, Wales and Ireland during the month of July. Of the 3069 cases completed, 2989 were found true, affecting the welfare of 8015 children and involving 3896 offenders. Warnings were issued in 2701 cases: 76 were prosecuted (resulting in 75 convictions): and 212 were dealt by transfer or in other ways. From its foundation in 1884 the Society has dealt with 1,033,453 complaints involving 2,906,706 children. In the Gateshead branch during the same month 14 cases were dealt with affecting 33 children. The local office of the Society is situated at 35, Bensham Road, Gateshead.

In the North Northumberland 17 cases were dealt with affecting 61 children, by the local office, 101, Newgate Street, Morpeth.

In the Newcastle branch 16 cases were dealt with, affecting 36 children, by the local office, 5 Guildford Place, Heaton."

Dr Cooper established good relations with the NSPCC which were maintained in later years by paediatricians concerned with Child Protection.

J.C. and his colleagues were well aware of the harmful effects of poor parental care, deprivation and defective social conditions on children in Newcastle, but the specific clinical involvement of paediatricians in the identification and management of physical and emotional abuse and neglect did not emerge until much later. The beginning of a greater understanding of the nature and extent of abuse and neglect in Newcastle is recorded in the 1000 Families Study of 1947.[18] This contains a brief chapter on 'Problem Families'. A rating scale of 30 possible 'deficiencies' was devised. Known and suspected cruelty and neglect were included, but no details are given [Table 25]. Out of 967 families visited throughout the first year of the study, 20 (2%) were rated as 'problem families'. Three kinds were identified, with appropriate case histories. The 'friendly', 'sullen' and 'vicious' kinds. The latter may be interpreted as a typical example of the Munchausen syndrome by proxy. The final comment in that case history is:

"By the time he was 4 months old, the mother was pregnant again."

The conclusions at the end of the chapter are of historical importance, because this was the first record in Newcastle of the recognition by paediatricians of an alarming and common problem regarding the health and welfare of children. J.C. and his colleagues appreciated the limitations of their assessment of families and the competency of a medical/paediatric intervention. Their conclusions are recorded in full, as they indicate the predicament of paediatricians during that era and how much had to be learnt and done to initiate an appropriate response:

"This limited assessment, however, gave no real idea of the baffling problem presented by these families both to their neighbours and to the numerous and generally uncoordinated social agencies who moved intermittently to their support but who rarely touched the heart of the problem. The basic defects of personality in most of the parents made wholesome family life impossible, and in the care of their children they needed supervision and support, based on an intimate knowledge of their defects. There has been no real improvement in these 20 families in the subsequent years of our survey, and we believe that by any scale applicable to English urban society they would represent the lowest level of family life.

The treatment of these 'problem families' cannot be considered here. It is clear that each community must acknowledge the problem, measure its size, analyse its component parts, and then through a firm partnership between public and voluntary service apply what remedies it can. The remedies will be preventive or palliative, for complete curative treatment may be impossible. We would suggest only that wise treatment is more likely to be reached by the methods of clinical scientists than by those of punitive empiricists. If the scientific method fails to supply an answer or provide a remedy, it would be best to rely on sentiments of charity and love. Finally we wish to suggest that in addition to probation officers, ministers, and other social workers who can come near to these 'problem families', family doctors, health visitors, district nurses, and home-helps might play a larger part."

Published by doctors in 1954, when knowledge about the identification of child abuse and neglect and the means of effective child protection involving health services were very limited, these comments already contain the seeds of the multi-disciplinary actions that eventually evolved in Newcastle as elsewhere in the country.

The historical background to the active involvement of the Babies Hospital in child protection may be traced back to shortly after 1951, when Dr Cooper assumed consultant responsibility for a group of young children at a residential nursery at Wellburn in rural Northumberland about twelve miles from Newcastle.[13]

The nursery at Ovingham opened in 1948, with an agreement at the time for ten of the 20 places to be occupied by Newcastle children in the care of the city's Children Department. These young children came from disordered 'problem families' or were infants awaiting adoption. These arrangements ceased in the early 1960s when the local authority places became available to the National Health Service. The nursery then became part of the Paediatric Department of Newcastle General Hospital and was staffed by nurses, nursery nurses and auxiliary nurses experienced in the care of young children. An increasing number were referred from severely disordered families in whom health, developmental or behavioural problems were also present. These children needed a period of good nutrition and care in addition to various medical treatments. They needed careful observation and assessment of their growth, development and behaviour and of their family problems. This was carried out by Dr Cooper and the staff in conjunction with the child psychiatry and psychology department, the social services and the community child health team. These children were largely deprived of love and care at home and a great deal of staff time was occupied in caring for them and in helping and encouraging their parents to continue improved care at home. Up to three mothers or other family members could stay in residence at any one time, caring for their children. As a result, a number of families were enabled to cope and avoid the need for their children to be taken into foster care. It was the forerunner of later special residential provisions for 'problem families' by paediatric services in a hospital setting in Newcastle, which began at the Babies Hospital at Leazes Terrace. The nursery also took in severely physically and mentally disabled children for long-term care or to give their family a break. It eventually closed in 1984.

During the 1960s, Dr Cooper arranged for the assessment at the Babies Hospital of a small number of selected infants with a view to adoption. There were two admissions for this purpose during the first six months of 1960 [Table 10]. This was the beginning of the hospital service concerned with child protection.

The weekly teaching sessions at the hospital for medical students, which had their origins in the demonstrations at West Parade by J.C. during the pre-war years, continued under Professor Court and other members of the Children's Department, notably Dr (later Professor) Michael Parkin [Figure 28]. They were very popular. By then, the medical students had been provided with a three month attachment to the paediatric wards of the main hospitals.

After the transfer of surgical services to the FMH, the number of children admitted to the Babies Hospital with infections and organic conditions decreased to less than 200 per year. The hospital closed in 1976. This became inevitable as paediatric sub-specialities developed and concentrated at the main hospitals in which provisions for resident mothers were by then more widely available. In 1972, the Ridley wing opened at the RVI with eight purpose-built cubicles for resident mothers and their children.

For 28 years, this Babies Hospital at Leazes Terrace had maintained the tradition, initiated by J.C., of the treatment of some of the youngest sick children of the community in an ambience distinct from that of the paediatric wards of the main hospitals, in which resident mothers could participate effectively in the nursing care of their sick babies and infants. Priorities evolved over the years and these included a service for young children with behaviour difficulties and others from 'problem families' with child protection issues during the final years of the hospital.

56

THE MOTHER AND CHILD UNIT
AT THE FLEMING MEMORIAL HOSPITAL FOR SICK CHILDREN
(FMH),
MARCH 1977 TO OCTOBER 1987

The value of the special services of the Babies Hospital was recognised and a limited provision of a residential facility for mothers and their children was provided at the FMH [Figure 29]. At the time, there was no imminent expectation for a new purpose-built children's hospital to include all the city's children inpatient services.

The decision to move to the FMH was a pragmatic one. A single ward consisting of seven cubicles capable of accommodating a mother and child became available following the closure of its gastroenteritis unit. The number and severity of the condition had been decreasing[63], in keeping with the decline of the disease in the community; a reduction already noted by J.C. in earlier years. The new unit was situated on the upper floor of the hospital away from the busy medical and surgical wards. The FMH was a famously friendly and popular children's hospital, which made the staff of the new unit very welcome. It was built in 1887 by Mr John Fleming in memory of his late wife. He was a local solicitor who also had interests in mining and a local colliery. The hospital replaced the original Children's Hospital in Hanover Square which was established in 1863 and closed in 1886.[15] In addition to the Mother and Child Unit, it contained a medical ward, the paediatric and plastic surgery services, a surgical neonatal intensive care unit, a children's burns ward and a specially adapted X-ray department. Parents were made welcome and separate accommodation, additional to the Mother and Child Unit was provided for them in lodgings nearby.

The first year (1977) was a transitional period when many surgical patients were admitted. Thereafter for a while, surgical admissions were for the purpose only of post-operative care. The details of the admissions over a representative number of years are shown in Tables 13, 14a and b, and Figure 31. Babies and young children under the age of 3 years figured prominently as at the Babies Hospital (53% in 1985), but a significant number of older children over the age of 5 years were also accommodated. Some had chronic medical conditions such as troublesome constipation and convulsions, but those over the age of ten years were children with severe physical and mental disabilities who came in on their own in order to give their families a period of relief as at the Wellburn Nursery in earlier years. It filled a gap in local services.

For a few years, a close link developed with the Special Care Baby Unit at the adjacent Princess Mary Maternity Hospital. Dr Edmund Hey, senior lecturer in Child Health, looked after his patients, whose mothers required a more extended period of help and support. As described in 1955 by Dr Leonard Strang, the ambience and facilities of a special hospital facility for resident mothers and babies may be well suited for the promotion of bonding and building up the confidence of the mother. This is of particular importance as there was increasing evidence that emotional deprivation, neglect and physical abuse were more prominent among low birth weight babies and others who needed to be in hospital during the newborn period.[64 and 65]

Amongst children with medical problems, there was a small group of special interest. These were toddlers with chronic constipation who, as was the case in 1985 [Table 14b], were admitted for a few days for further investigation and support of the mothers. Some required a manual removal under anaesthesia and a rectal biopsy. There was a history of anal fissure in a few but no other specific organic causes were found. The condition also caused a great deal of distress for their parents. Some had been referred by the paediatric surgeons. A special outpatient follow-up clinic was set up. This led to an important study of the bowel habit of young children.[66] It was conducted by Dr Lawrence Weaver, the paediatric registrar at the Fleming Hospital. The study was undertaken in a well-defined community in one general practice in the suburban new town of Cramlington in Northumberland. Dr Weaver was already responsible for a Child Health Clinic in that practice as part of his paediatric training, a service in which J.C. himself had been involved in Newcastle shortly before he was appointed Honorary Medical Officer to the West End Day Nursery in 1923. Dr Weaver later succeeded to the Chair of Paediatrics at Glasgow University. Up to that time, normative data about bowel function had not been available anywhere for children between the ages of 1 and 4 years.

The changes that had taken place at the Babies Hospital during 1976 with the admission of children from families with 'social problems' were consolidated. Compared with 20% of all admissions in 1976, the average from four representative years was 63% rising to 93% during 1987. These included a number of children with medical conditions from families with 'social problems'. The remainder were from families with significant issues of child protection, in whom poor care, abuse and neglect had already been detected or a high risk of harm identified. The proportion of this vulnerable group rose to 75% of all admissions in 1987.

As a result, the Mother and Child Unit at the FMH came to specialise in the assessment of babies and young children from vulnerable 'problem families' who were not acutely ill, in contrast to the preponderance of life threatening medical and surgical emergencies of earlier years and the more chronic organic disorders at the Babies Hospital at Leazes Terrace [Figure 30]. By 1985, 64% of the children were admitted with their mothers, rising to 96% in 1987

A series of case histories from the report of "The Mother and Child Unit. 1977-1985"[13] illustrates the different problems that were encountered. This report was written from a paediatric perspective with the specific intention of publicising the history and the work of the Unit in order to make a 'case of need' for the relocation of the service on a suitable site and environment with the imminent closure of the Fleming Hospital. This accounts for the inclusion of detailed administrative arrangements and the description of the multidisciplinary nature of the work. There was also an attempt to justify the validity of the continued involvement of hospital based paediatricians and nurses in the continuation of the service in this special area of child protection, at a time when community services were beginning to undertake this work.

The decade before the closure of the Fleming Hospital was punctuated with concerns by paediatricians and all those actively involved in child care about the best way of dealing with suspected abuse and neglect. There was always the possibility of a mistaken diagnosis with disastrous consequences for the families and the professionals concerned. Expertise and multidisciplinary systems of management were still developing. The Fleming Unit played a useful part in the management of the problem during that era. As far as it was known at the time, this was the only residential paediatric hospital service in the country undertaking this kind of work.

Until her retirement in 1983, Dr Cooper was responsible for most of the children with child protection issues. The first admission to the unit under her care of a newborn baby at high risk of harm at the hands of her parents occurred in the middle of 1979. It paved the way for future attempts to safeguard newborn babies and support their families. It gives an indication of the considerable difficulties involved and the need during that era for paediatric services in a hospital setting to acquire new areas of expertise in order to attempt a useful contribution.

Miss E. Greenacre, who was a staff nurse (and later senior sister) at the Mother and Child Unit at the time, clearly recalls the circumstances, as they were such a considerable cause of controversy. The baby was the first child of a young mother and it was realised during the pregnancy that her partner had a previous family in which two of his children had sustained non-accidental injuries; one was seriously damaged. The father was responsible. The mother had no knowledge of her partner's previous history and was unwilling to give up her relationship with him. The baby was made a Ward of Court and the social services wanted to remove the baby into foster care at birth.

Dr Cooper was asked by the court to make an assessment of the family and the baby was admitted with her mother from the maternity hospital to the FMH within a few days of birth. She settled well. The father visited regularly under supervision. Dr Cooper spent a great deal of time with the parents and the staff did their best to provide guidance and support. In the event, after several weeks of observation and support and much heart-searching, the baby was allowed to go home to the care of the parents. The decision was made in conjunction with the social services and the approval of the court. The family did well at least in the short term. There is no information about later outcome, but there was no news from the community social and health services about a breakdown of care or harm to the child. This would undoubtedly have come to the notice of Dr Cooper and the staff of the hospital over the following four years before her retirement.

At the outset, a new set of nursing staff was appointed. This included a senior sister, two staff nurses and several auxiliaries. A full-time nursery nurse, Miss Christine Cardose, was also appointed and made an invaluable contribution to the service over the next twenty years. Initially, the experience of the staff was limited. It increased rapidly with the frequent regular contacts with

59

Dr Cooper, who spent a considerable part of her time in discussions about the children from families with social problems and in training the staff [Figure 31].

The experience of participating in increasing numbers of multi-disciplinary case conferences was also of vital importance, as was the fact that the senior staff held together over the years to become skilled in the assessment and support of vulnerable children and their families. At the end of 1985, fathers, siblings and other family members were also taken in with the mothers. The name was changed to the Family Unit.

When Dr Cooper retired in 1983, one of the authors of this study of J.C.'s legacy, Dr Hans Steiner (H.S.) took over clinical responsibility for the Unit and most children, including those from families with 'social problems', came under his care. He was senior lecturer in child health and a consultant paediatrician in Newcastle and Northumberland. As well as an association with Dr Cooper for several years, there had been extensive training and experience in the assessment of growth and development,[67] clinical experience in the diagnosis of child abuse and neglect and in the field of social paediatrics.[68]

Special arrangements had to be made for the families with issues of child protection. Following a referral from health services, social services or the NSPCC, preliminary home visits were undertaken by H.S. with a social worker or occasionally the family's health visitor. The full-time hospital social worker, Miss Sue Jackson, took part in some of these visits during the early years. Later, the community social worker was involved. Case conferences on a multi-disciplinary basis were sometimes convened before admission to the Unit. This preparation was intended to gather all the available information from health and social services, whose records were usually made available. The home visits were arranged to gain some insight into the conditions there, as well as a first step in gaining the confidence of parents. This was reinforced for some of them by visits to the hospital, which introduced them to members of the staff who explained the daily routines and the arrangements for their assessment and support. Some parents had unhappy experiences with health services in the past and some had been traumatised in court during legal proceedings for the protection of their children. Considerable reassurance was sometimes required.

A vital addition to the assessment of 'problem families' was the involvement of psychologists and child psychiatrists from the Nuffield Unit for Children and Young People, conveniently located in the grounds of the Fleming Memorial Hospital.

Dr Cooper initiated these arrangements at the Wellburn Nursery during the early 1950s and later at the Babies Hospital at Leazes Terrace. These arrangements were extended at the FMH to include an increasing number of families.

The paediatric assessment, allied to that of the nursing staff and nursery nurse, was designed to record the strength of the attachment of the mother (and later other family members or caretakers) to the child, the quality of care, the health, growth, development and behaviour of the child, and the progress that was made in the provision of care. The ability and willingness of the mother to learn and cooperate with the staff and her ability to relate to her partner and other families resident on the unit were also assessed.

60

The assessments by the child psychologists and child psychiatrists were concerned with the intellectual abilities and educational attainments of the parents, their personalities and tolerance to the stresses of their lives, family function, and risk factors in their daily life and social environment.

Assessments of the children's progress were made and adult psychiatrists were sometimes involved to assess the parents. Mothers with acute or significant chronic psychiatric illness were admitted elsewhere at times with their babies, to psychiatric hospitals.

Although the hospital social worker took part in some of the assessments, the community social worker remained the 'key worker' and continued to assess the social and environmental conditions of the family and their ability and willingness to cooperate with the community services. The hospital assessments were completed in most cases in a period of about four weeks. The facilities and resources of the Mother and Child Unit were not suited to a more prolonged stay. However, a longer period was sometimes required when mothers needed to spend some time at home for a break and to sort out their affairs. It was the firm view of all concerned that the value of such a relatively short period of hospital residence in a safe environment, as part of a multidisciplinary assessment, was appropriate specifically for babies and infants.

A multi-disciplinary case conference was convened at the conclusion of the assessment, when recommendations were made about the future care of the child and what help and support might be required. A comprehensive paediatric report, as well as an independent one by the psychologist and child psychiatrist, was written on discharge. This had to be suitable for court proceedings when necessary and additional meetings with legal representatives had sometimes to be arranged. An indication of the magnitude of the work is the thirty-one conferences attended during 1985 by the nursing staff and nursery nurse and the sixty-three attended by the consultant paediatrician.

During the decade of the life of the Mother and Child Unit from 1988 when the work of the Unit had settled into a routine, 483 children were admitted from families with issues of child protection. They represented 35.5% of all the admissions to the unit up to 1987. These data are recorded in the Report from the Family Unit of 1991 under the heading of "psycho-social" problems, the nomenclature adopted during that era.[14] In 1985, fathers, partners and siblings were admitted and the name was changed to The Family Unit.

The courts by then were also supportive; the days when magistrates in Newcastle expressed their antagonism towards paediatricians and others who engaged with and supported these vulnerable families had long gone. This was in part due to the example of a dispassionate yet humane approach by Dr Cooper and the staff of the Mother and Child Unit at the FMH, who demonstrated that support and help could be successfully provided for some of these troubled families.

A review of the short-term outcome was made in the 64 children from 49 'problem families' admitted over a two-year period from 1984 to 1985 (Table 15): 49 (77%) were discharged home after the period of residential assessment. The remainder (15) went into foster care; three on a voluntary basis. About one year later, five (10%) of the 49 originally discharged home were taken into foster care

61

following a breakdown in parental care. Fortunately none had been physically abused or seriously neglected

These preliminary findings were presented to the Psychiatry and Psychology Group at the Annual Scientific Meeting of the British Paediatric Association in 1986.[69]

The long-term outcome was uncertain. The responsibility weighed heavily on everyone concerned at the hospital. Life-changing recommendations were being made at considerable risk. Nevertheless, it was possible to support and help some of these 'problem families', even some with the most extreme disadvantages. It was likely during that era in Newcastle and the northern region, that some would have been taken into foster care permanently with a view to adoption, especially newborn babies 'at risk', in the absence of the kind of residential assessment and support that was available at the Mother and Child Unit.

Education

The teaching sessions with medical students did not continue. However, senior house officers, paediatric registrars and student nurses had experience at the Unit and a great deal was learned by everyone attending case conferences. This experience was communicated to other services. Numerous lectures were given by H.S., the nursery nurse and the senior sister to primary care services, postgraduate doctors, hospital staff, medical students, nurses and nursery nurses in training, midwives, education services and social workers, on the identification, assessment and management of child abuse and neglect.

The closure of the Fleming Hospital in 1987

There was no longer a requirement for the medical ward and the surgical services were also transferred to the RVI. Much more appropriate facilities for intensive care and technical investigations were available there and close proximity to paediatric sub-specialities was a significant advantage. Financial considerations came into play. A case of need was accepted for the continuation of the services of the Mother and Child Unit. The Unit was transferred, with all the nursing staff and nursery nurse, to the grounds of Newcastle General Hospital in a building separate to the paediatric wards of that hospital.

J.C.'s legacy of a special hospital provision for babies and infants had been maintained and evolved to meet new challenges and priorities that had emerged in paediatric practice. In addition, paediatricians accompanied by nursing staff ventured into the community, as he had intended when he maintained that hospital doctors should work in the community from time to time as "field workers" to study the prevalent diseases.[97]

Case Histories

The Mother and Child Unit, Fleming Hospital. 1978 – 1987
Transcribed from "The Mother and Child Unit, The Fleming Hospital. History, development and use."[13]

A. Medical condition. Obesity

Age 4 years
Admitted with father

B. Medical condition (dermatitis)
with social problems

Age 6 weeks

Issues of child protection

C. Neglect and non-accidental
injuries

Age 4 months
To foster care

D. Failure to thrive

Age 10 months
Discharged home

E. Newborn baby with mother

Age 12 days
To foster care

F. Problems of care, family
dysfunction and strife

Age 10 months
Discharged home

G. Unstable family with chronic
psychiatric problems and violent father

Age 4 months
Discharged home

H. Suspected physical abuse

Age 20 months
No evidence of abuse
Discharged home

I. Sexual abuse

Age 12 years
Back to Care Home

J.   Severe   physical   and   mental
disability

Age 11 years.
Respite care

K.   Severe   physical   and   mental
disability with convulsions. Parents no
longer able to cope at home

Age 9 months
**Discharged to foster
care**

Family A. At age 4 years and 3 months, this child had gross obesity with a weight of 28.9 Kg (well above the 97th centile). Her height was on the 75th centile and there were no other abnormal physical findings. She was however very slow and clumsy and would not take a normal active part in school activities. She was originally referred to H.S. at a paediatric outpatient clinic in Berwick in Northumberland and then admitted to the Fleming Unit for further assessment and dieting. Originally it had been arranged for her mother to come in and stay with her, but the family insisted that the father should come instead.

The investigations excluded an endocrine and definable metabolic abnormality and we came to the conclusion that the problem was due to a combination of genetic and family factors. Her mother, who is 46 years of age, is also grossly obese and so are several members of her family. Her father, who is 52 years, is also much overweight. She is the youngest, by far, of a family of 4 children, (her siblings being 20, 22 and 24 years old) and she had clearly been overindulged. The eating habits of the family were totally unsatisfactory. We learnt that the father could not work because of recurrent problems with rheumatoid arthritis.

During the six days stay at the hospital, she was started on a diet of 900 calories per day on the advice of a dietician. Her father also joined in and decided to try and lose weight. He became interested in the whole process. He took her out regularly for walks to Exhibition Park nearby. She lost 800 grams during her stay. On returning home, she continued to do well. Her weight six months later was just above the 97th centile. She became much more agile and relatives and friends and her teachers at school commented on her greatly increased liveliness and a much more outgoing personality.

Her father continued to take charge of her diet and had insisted on changing routines at home in order to help her. He also lost weight, but to his chagrin not very much. Her mother readily concurred with the new arrangements.

Comment

This child could have been admitted to an ordinary paediatric ward with resident parent accommodation. However it would not have been possible to provide the required privacy, flexibility and atmosphere of calm support that enabled her father to settle down rapidly and acquire the confidence and skill to effect a major change in this child's life.

Family B. Age 6 weeks. Referred by a consultant paediatrician from the RVI, where he had been admitted six days before. His mother had taken him to the Casualty Department because of a severe nappy rash, which was spreading over his trunk. She claimed to have phoned her family doctor requesting a home visit but none had been forthcoming.

Both the mother and child were admitted to a paediatric ward of the RVI, where his thrush was treated. It was quickly evident that there were many other problems. Mother aged 21 years is single and has another child aged 2 years. The father comes from Pakistan and has a family of his own. He visits regularly but provides little help and support. Mother felt exhausted and unable to cope with her two children. She has slapped her and was afraid of doing her real harm.

A consultation with a psychiatrist was arranged at the RVI. Although there were some signs of depression and anxiety, a diagnosis of a formal psychiatric illness was not appropriate. It was felt that there were many adverse personality, family and social factors affecting the family and that a further period of assessment and treatment in the Fleming Mother and Child Unit might be beneficial.

The baby turned out to have a very sensitive skin with severe seborrhaeic dermatitis as well as thrush. He had diarrhoea and evidence of intolerance to cow's milk, which responded to a switch to soya milk. His mother expressed a great deal of anxiety about his skin problem because of a fear that he might have eczema (the child's father has this problem) and she required considerable reassurance, which only proved successful when his skin improved.

We offered to accommodate her other child on the Unit, but this offer was not taken up as she was already cared for by the maternal grandmother. The psychiatrist continued to see her and confirmed the absence of any psychiatric illness. The baby was thriving and developing normally.

It was clear that the mother would require additional help and support and a case conference was held at the Day Nursery in the east end of Newcastle which the 2 year old sibling had been attending on a fulltime basis for some time. The staff of the Nursery knew the family very well and it was felt to be the most appropriate site for a conference.

The consultant paediatrician (H.S.), staff nurse and the nursery nurse from the Unit attended together with the hospital social worker, who had taken a major part in the assessment of the family.

Although a great deal was already known about the family by the health visitor and the nursery staff, it was useful to pool information to see how best to help and support the family in the future. Mother was to be encouraged to spend more time at the Nursery with her two children and the local area social services Team was to be asked to provide further social work support. (A representative of the Team was invited to attend the case conference but could not do so at the last minute). A clear commitment was made by the primary health care team to monitor the children's health and progress on a regular basis, as it was felt inappropriate for the family to return to the hospital for this purpose.

The family was discharged home after 19 days on the Unit. Mother felt much better, was a lot less anxious and more confident in coping with the baby's care.

Comment

The ambience of the Fleming Unit was more suited to helping this family than a busy paediatric ward. A multidisciplinary approach was taken, involving psychiatrists, hospital social worker, health visitor and Nursery staff. The flexible working arrangements are well illustrated by the ready availability of the senior hospital staff to go out into the community when appropriate.

Family C. Age 4 months. He was transferred to the Fleming Unit from Sunderland following a joint referral by a paediatrician and social worker. He had been admitted ten weeks earlier to the local District General Hospital in a grossly neglected state and unwell with a urinary tract infection. During the course of the admission to the hospital, two fractured ribs had been found on x-ray. The mother's cohabitee had admitted to the police that he had 'hugged' the baby hard on at least one occasion.

It was clear that the mother required a great deal of advice and help with the baby's care. An Interim Care Order had already been obtained and the purpose of the admission to the Fleming Unit was to determine whether his mother (age 23) could be taught to look after him adequately and whether he could then safely be returned home.

From the outset it was clear that there were appalling problems. His mother's life had been most unhappy and disturbed. Her parent's marriage was unstable and they eventually divorced. Her father obtained custody of the children (all six of them) and they all lived under poor conditions. Eventually she went into Care (as did her five siblings) and was away from home most of her early life. She had been sexually assaulted by her father and elder brother on several occasions before the age of 17. She had most of her schooling at a special residential (ESN/M) school where she made little progress. During the pregnancy she had severe anaemia, but failed to cooperate with treatment and on one occasion discharged herself from hospital against medical advice. She had already lost one baby at the age of two days with pneumonia.

Less was known about the mother's boyfriend (age 21 and unemployed). It was not certain that he was the father of the child. He was brought up by his grandmother and was placed on a Care Order at the age of 14 for arson. He also had several convictions for assault and wounding and other minor offences. He was apparently due to appear in court for cruelty to a dog.

Although the mother and her partner had been together for two years, there had been a considerable amount of discord. There was little support from the extended family. The boyfriend's father was registered blind, was mentally disabled and had a conviction for sexual assault. Mother had indicated to the social worker that it would be best for the baby to go into Care, and it is strongly suspected that the reason is that her boyfriend needs her to look after him. The families were well known to the local social services department over many years because of multiple difficulties.

During the child's stay on the Unit, it became abundantly clear that his mother was attached to him, loved him, but could not provide him with the consistent basic care required for safe health and appropriate growth and development. The detailed observations of the nursing staff and nursery nurse showed that the mother required repeated prompting and reminding in the preparation of feeds, which she failed to learn to do adequately. She needed constant help with changing and bathing and reminders to do so when the baby needed it. She was often forgetful and failed to anticipate his needs.

He was a contented baby who was generally easy to handle, but when unsettled, mother was unable to settle him because she simply did not have the patience to do so. Her needs (e.g. watching TV) generally came first. A psychological assessment by a clinical psychologist from the Nuffield Child Psychiatry Unit confirmed her limited abilities and educational attainments.

The mother's boyfriend was extremely reluctant to visit, despite the special arrangement to pay his fares and the offer of overnight accommodation. He was eventually persuaded to come into residence on the Unit, but stayed only three days. It was clear that he was not interested in the baby and was reluctant to handle him. Despite much encouragement, he did not provide any of the basic care. The relationship with the baby's mother was unstable. They bickered all day long about everyday matters including the care of the baby. It was not possible, in the limited time available, for him to have a formal psychological assessment, but it was also evident that he had limited abilities. The baby had apparently been left in his care from time to time and although there was no direct evidence, it is likely that the baby's injuries could well have been caused in moments of frustration.

The baby thrived but there were already indications of impaired development in that his social responses (e.g. smiling) were limited, especially when his mother was looking after him. She simply was not 'synchronised' with him.

Three weeks after his admission, it was decided at a case conference that he could not safely be returned home and that any further period of assessment and teaching would not be productive and not in his best interest. He was discharged to foster parents and a full Care Order was obtained.

At the age of six months, he was doing very well and was now developing and responding normally in foster care.

Comment

The assessment revealed the early signs of failure to progress so far as the social responses were concerned. It was clear that the mother could not care safely for him despite a great deal of help and support and that she did not have any family support. The attempt at rehabilitation was terminated in the best interests of the child because it was felt that no further progress was possible.

Family D. At 10 months was failing to thrive as a result of inadequate care at home. It was estimated that she was receiving only half the calories per day for normal growth.

Her mother was single, 26 years old and of limited abilities. She did not feed her consistently despite considerable support from her heath visitor and community social worker.

She began to thrive during the six weeks of residence in the Mother and Child Unit. The mother was strongly attached to her and responded readily to the support and advice of the nursing staff and nursery nurse.

Her skills improved and progress was maintained at home. Further help and supervision were arranged with her heath visitor and community social worker.

Comment

As at the Babies Hospital, the ambience and experience of the nursing staff and nursery nurse were well suited to the purpose of helping and supporting this at a time when the baby's progress was delayed despite maximum available support in the community.

Family E. Age 12 days when admitted to the Fleming Unit from the postnatal ward of Ashington Hospital in Northumberland. The purpose of the admission was to make an assessment of the parents' motivation and ability to care for him and to teach and support them to do so effectively. Their first child had been taken into Care when he was a few months old because of their inability to care for him, despite extensive and intense community help.

His mother had a very unhappy and deprived childhood; she had been in Care herself. She had an immature personality and was of limited intelligence. She also had a history of unstable behaviour and violence and had tried to commit suicide soon after the child's birth. His father was also known to have limited abilities and went to a special ESN(M) school. He was an epileptic and drunk heavily. The material and environmental standards had always been poor.

The decision to try and help the family to care for their new baby was taken in consultation with their social worker, health visitor and family doctor. It was felt that the relationship between the couple was more stable. They had married, she had maintained that they had made attempts to improve their living conditions and they were cooperating well with all the primary health care and social services. They visited the Unit, met the staff and readily agreed to come in.

Mother was resident. Father visited regularly and took an active part in the care of the baby. Breastfeeding was established and with training and supervision, good basic care was established. Both parents were well attached to their child and appeared to get on well together. They all went home after a stay of two weeks. Intensive community support and supervision were set up.

The baby did well over the next few months, growing and developing normally, but the relationship between the parents deteriorated and they separated when the child was about 2 years of age. At that point, the mother moved from Northumberland to Newcastle to live with her mother. She eventually moved into her own flat.

By the time the child reached the age of 2 years and 10 months, his mother was finding it very difficult to cope with his very disturbed behaviour. He often had temper tantrums and screaming attacks and she found it virtually impossible to control him. He was attending a Day Nursery, where his behaviour was much improved, but he then relapsed at home.

They were both readmitted to the Fleming Unit. He was a well grown healthy child and we were able to observe the extremely negative behaviour towards his mother, his temper tantrums, failure to feed properly, lack of toilet training and sleep disturbances.

She found it quite impossible to manage, despite a great deal of help and support. She would very easily give up and leave it to the staff, who were able without much difficulty to obtain appropriate responses from him. In fact he behaved quite reasonably in mother's absence and proved to be a very inquisitive little boy, who was keen to learn. We found his mother to be a very unhappy and unsettled lady and it became clear that not only was she unable to care for him adequately, but she was unwilling to do so, She told us that everything went reasonably well during the first six months of his life, but then she began to resent the demands that he was making on her and felt that she did not have a life of her own. These feelings increased particularly when the relationship with her husband deteriorated. It became clear that his disturbed behaviour was related to his mother's lack of warmth and feeling towards him.

During their stay, the hospital social worker took part in the assessment and much effort was put into trying to help this lady over a period of seven weeks.

A psychological assessment by a clinical psychologist from the Nuffield Child Psychiatry Unit showed her to have abilities at the lower end of normal, with relatively good education attainments, particularly reading. She was certainly capable of understanding her child's needs and had the ability to learn new skills and bring up a family.

She was a very lonely person, with no recreational outlets. It became clear that she was no longer willing to look after her child and arrangements were made for him to go into foster care on a voluntary basis.

Her relief to be able to express her feelings and to know that alternative care was possible for her child were very evident. She was not at any time clinically depressed. Over the next few months in foster care, he did very well and his behaviour improved considerably.

Comment

Even with the establishment of a good bond between mother and child in the newborn period and the early months of life, the outcome was a 'disaster' for the family and potentially for the child.

Ultimately the mother did not have the personal resources, or the family support, to care for him.

It illustrates the need for follow up of progress over a long period of time in order to assess the value to the child of the work of the Unit. It will be interesting to determine the outcome amongst the newborn babies discharged home this year following a period of assessment, teaching and help.

Family F. Age 10 months. His mother, age 19, arrived at the Fleming Unit with him quite unexpectedly. There had been a domestic dispute with violence to her by her boyfriend (also aged 19). The police had been called and she was afraid that he would harm the baby. She had no money and there was no food in the house.

She came to us because she thought that we would be sympathetic to her, following an admission three months before, when the child had a mild gastro-enteritis and she derived much benefit from an admission to the Unit at a time when he was very fretful and she was unable to cope at home. She was adamant in her refusal to seek help from her community social worker, who knew her well, because of her fear of having the baby removed, and unwilling to go to the 'battered wives' hostel in Newcastle.

She stayed for four days, during which time contact was made with the health visitor and social worker to arrange further support and supervision. The child was well and progressing normally except for a tendency to fretfulness.

Family G. Age 4 months. He was admitted as an emergency following a referral by a social worker from The Family Service Unit in Newcastle. A crisis had occurred at home following the return of her cohabitee after his discharge from a psychiatric hospital, where he had been treated for relapse of schizophrenia. The social worker felt that he presented a danger to the baby because of his instability and liability to violence, especially when under the influence of alcohol. Also, the mother finds it 'impossible' to live on her own. She herself is on treatment for schizophrenia, which is well controlled at present, but she does get very anxious on her own and then cannot cope with the baby. The present crisis was compounded by the fact that she had fallen out with her sister, with whom she had been staying.

The social worker felt that she needed somewhere safe to stay, where support and help were available, whilst further help was arranged. There was no place at the social services' Family Care Centre at Ryehill in Newcastle. She did in fact spend a night there the previous day, but could not be accommodated further. There was the further complication that neither the mother (nor her cohabitee) would agree to stay at this centre. She had been there with her previous baby five years ago, but was transferred within a few days to a psychiatric hospital, with a recurrence of her illness. This baby is now adopted.

She had up to now coped with her child with a lot of community support. The baby was healthy and progressing normally. They stayed on the Unit for ten days. During this time she settled down and was persuaded to go and live in sheltered accommodation, which was arranged during her admission to the Fleming. The social worker discussed the relationship with her boyfriend (who is the father of the child). As a result the mother decided to live by herself with the help that was being mobilised in the community. This included a placement conveniently nearby at a Day Nursery, where mother could also join in the activities. Continuing intensive social work, health visitor supervision and support were arranged.

It is interesting to note that there had already been contact with the Fleming Unit during her pregnancy. It was suggested that the mother might benefit from a stay there to help her gain confidence and learn to look after the baby. It was also felt that she had 'matured' considerably during the last five years, since her first pregnancy and would probably now be able to cope. She visited the Unit before the birth but declined to come afterwards.

Comment

The admission of these two families illustrates one function of the Mother and Child Unit – that is to be part of the network for families in trouble. It is arguable whether a paediatric input is appropriate. Nevertheless, we were able to safeguard the welfare of these children and ensure that their health and development would not be impaired. For some families, a health facility may be more acceptable than one from social services, because of the stigma attached to the latter in that era and fear of removal by the social services department of the children into Care.

In both these cases, the children remained with the mother because they appeared to be doing reasonably well despite the chaos and the strife. In other cases, health, growth and development may be impaired and paediatricians are in a definitive position to advise social services about the effects on children of adverse family and social conditions.

Family H. At 20 months was admitted with her mother following a referral by her family doctor in consultation with the practice health visitor and a social worker from the local area social services department. Child abuse was suspected. Some bruises were found on the child's face by the health visitor, who happened to visit the home of the child minder who was looking after her, whilst her mother (age 26) was working as a part time cleaner. The father (age 24) was in full employment as an electrical technician.

The health visitor contacted the social services department and the mother readily agreed to have the child examined in the Day Unit of a paediatric department in Newcastle, where they were taken by the social worker.

After an interview by the paediatric registrar on duty and a thorough examination, it was decided that this was not a case of non-accidental injuries. There had been major feeding difficulties and the bruising was thought to have been caused by forced feeding. The child went home the same day.

Three days later, following a follow up visit by the health visitor, further bruising was noted. The health visitor again contacted the social services department and in consultation with the family doctor, a referral was made to the Fleming Unit for a further assessment.

The child was well. Her general growth and development were entirely normal. There was bruising on the cheeks entirely compatible with finger tip pressure marks.

The history that was obtained was clear, consistent and entirely believable. This was a normal family who had made adequate preparation and provision for their child. She was a planned and wanted baby. The pregnancy, labour and delivery at term were all normal. From birth, she had been a very fretful baby, presenting considerable feeding difficulties (by bottle), a tendency to vomiting and a great deal of crying. She was not a cuddly baby and mother found it difficult to settle her down.

There is no clear cut explanation for the baby's abnormal behaviour. She was planned and wanted and both parents said that they were delighted with her. Her mother was well during the early months of pregnancy and in particular not unduly tired or depressed. There were no indications of drug abuse during the pregnancy. It may be that inexperience played an important part. Very soon feeding became a battle, so that by now she often stored food in her mouth and was 'force fed' in desperation. Mother had frequently sought advice from the health visitor and local Child Health Clinic but the situation had failed to improve.

There was further deterioration when the child was 6 months of age, when the mother had an acute asthma attack for the first time in her life, which frightened her badly. By the time they were admitted to the Mother and Child Unit, the family was fraught, bewildered and afraid of losing their child, particularly as a child of the mother's sister had been taken into Care following abuse.

During their six days stay on the Unit, we were able to confirm that apart from severe feeding difficulties, the child was normal, well attached to her mother and father and that there were no adverse family and social conditions. She was by all accounts happy and settled with the child minder.

Simple straightforward advice by the nursing staff produced a marked improvement. The family settled and were reassured. Three months later, the child was progressing well at home and all feeding difficulties had disappeared.

Comment
This was a problem of inappropriate childcare and not child abuse. The initial paediatric assessment suggested the diagnosis but the consultation was limited to the exclusion of child abuse. A short stay in the Mother and Child Unit resolved the problem. It illustrates the need of a comprehensive paediatric assessment in suspected child abuse, which is not limited to a diagnosis of bruises, but includes an expert assessment of growth and development, and the family and social factors that may have an adverse effect.

A residential assessment may at times be necessary to resolve these kinds of difficulties. The ambience of the Fleming Unit was well suited to helping this family. The close links and mutual respect that had developed over the years with the social services department of the area in which the family lives, enabled us to arrive at a rapid and satisfactory conclusion so far as the family were concerned and avoid further lengthy child abuse investigations as set out in the guidelines for the management of these cases.

Family I. Age 12 years. Admitted from a Family Group Home. She had been sexually abused by her father during an access visit. A vaginal trichomonas infection was detected and treated. Joint care with a child psychiatrist and a community social worker was arranged.

Family J. Age 11 years. Severe physical and mental disability (cerebral palsy). Admitted in order to give his mother a break from the arduous care that he required at home. Her husband was often away at sea for long periods of time. Respite care facilities in the city were limited at that time.

Family K. Age 9 months. Severe physical and mental disability following birth trauma. He required a great deal of nursing care at home and had frequent convulsions. The family could not cope any longer to look after him. They were introduced to a foster mother whilst at the Fleming Unit and were awaiting discharge to her home.

NOTE: Separate independent reports from the psychologists and psychiatrists were available when they participated in the assessments.

THE FAMILY UNIT
AT NEWCASTLE GENERAL HOSPITAL 1988 - 1997

The service continued with a further development in the assessment and support of families with 'social problems'. By 1990, they made up the bulk of the admissions apart from the group of children with severe physical and mental disabilities who came to give their families some relief [Tables 13, 16, 17 and Figure 30].

A distinction was made between families who required solely a period of observation, support and treatment to assist them in the care of their children and those referred specifically for an assessment about future care. Some of the former had medical conditions that also required attention; the average length of stay of ten days reflected the less demanding nature of their problems [Table 16]. The remainder who came for a family assessment had serious child protection issues. They required a longer period of residence of an average of 6-8 weeks. Many of their children were already in foster care on protection orders and permission was granted from the courts in order to assist social services to determine whether a return home with continuing support was appropriate. It was in these cases that the concept of 'good-enough parenting' promoted by Dr Cooper in earlier years[62] contributed greatly to the recommendations.

The most significant change in clinical practice during the life of this Family Unit was the increase in the involvement of child psychology and psychiatry in the assessments. For three years after 1994, this applied to all families when the Nuffield Child Psychiatry Unit in Newcastle took over full responsibility for the Family Unit.

Fathers or partners and siblings were now admitted. During 1988 to 1 April 1991, amongst a total of 148 children from families with 'social problems', 45% were accompanied by mother only, 40% by both parents or caretakers and 14% by a sibling and parent(s). Only two children were admitted on their own for observation. So far as the families with issues of child protection were concerned during 1988 to 1 April 1991, 81 (69%) out of 117 children admitted specifically for assessment of their parents' and caretakers' ability to provide safe and appropriate care for them were allowed to go home following a recommendation of a multidisciplinary case conference and with the permission of the courts where appropriate [Table 17]. This compares with a higher proportion allowed home (77%) immediately after the assessment of the 49 families admitted to the Mother and Child Unit at the Fleming Hospital during 1984-1985 [Table 15].

There was a strong impression of a marked increase in the complexities and high risks associated with these cases. This is borne out by a decrease in the proportion allowed to be cared for by their family at home and the breakdowns in the assessments in later years due to the disruptive behaviour of some of the parents and partners (see below). It was also apparent that the proceedings in court, especially in Wardship cases, became more difficult and

73

adversarial as complexities increased. Nevertheless, it was reassuring that the recommendations to allow the child to go home after assessment were almost always accepted by the courts. Between 1988 and 1 April 1991, there were only two occasions when the courts did not accept recommendations for rehabilitation. In both cases, it concerned children at high risk of harm, who had sustained multiple non-accidental fractures in the first 3 months of life.

The case histories from the report of 1991 from the Family Unit illustrate the severity and multiple deprivations that were often encountered.[14] By comparison with the case histories from the Mother and Child Unit of the Fleming Hospital compiled six years earlier in 1985, these accounts were intended primarily to record the nature of the problems of the families and changes that took place after the service transferred to the Family Unit at Newcastle General Hospital, rather than a 'case of need' for the continued provision of the service. This is reflected in the contents, which no longer include the reasons for the continuation of the service and how the service operated. The emphasis is on the clinical, family and social details and the outcome. The contents include the principal paediatric and nursing contributions, including that of the nursery nurse. These summaries were written by H.S. and formed the basis of the paediatric reports that were usually presented to the courts. There was close collaboration and discussions with the psychologist and child psychiatrists who produced their own independent reports. On reading these accounts again after an interval of 23 years, there is a striking uniformity about the distressing past histories of nearly all these families and the 'cycle of deprivation' that is revealed.

Non-accidental injuries – fractures and bruising in infants

A particularly challenging group of children was identified because of the exceptional difficulties and high risks involved. These were infants under the age of 12 months, with most less than 3 months of age, with non-accidental fractures and varying degrees of bruising. During a period of 13 years, starting at the Mother and Child Unit at the Fleming Hospital in 1978, up to 1 April 1991 at the Family Unit at Newcastle General Hospital, 26 infants had been admitted for a family assessment with their mother and later with fathers or partners [Tables 18 and 19]. Some of the early cases had been under the care of Dr Cooper. A firm diagnosis of non-accidental injuries had been made during the initial admission to a paediatric ward elsewhere in Newcastle and the northern region. The police had interviewed the families and the social services were involved with a legal responsibility for the child. All the children were already in foster care or with other family members including grandparents. Some parents had been prosecuted and three fathers had been jailed.

Eighteen (69%) were rehabilitated home with the consent of the courts. Eight were returned to foster care with a view to eventual adoption. After an average period of 16 months (range 4 to 51 months), two children who had been returned home were subsequently abused again, albeit not severely injured (and no fractures). One child was neglected and one sustained further bruises. One of the eight infants initially discharged into foster care was allowed home two months later.

By the time the Family Unit was involved and despite the obvious risks of further harm to all these children, a return to the family home was to be considered. It was the nature of the violence in such very young children that suggested an added significant risk of further harm. There was at the time, a willingness in some quarters to keep an open mind about the prospects of rehabilitation, even in severe high risk situations. At the Family Unit in Newcastle, this was mainly the result of the teachings and inspiration of Dr Cooper. She suggested that the maturity of parents and the family circumstances could improve sufficiently to provide safe and 'good-enough parenting' in some cases even in very vulnerable families, provided that they received the right support, help and supervision.

Some preliminary findings were presented to a scientific meeting of the Psychiatry and Psychology Group at the Annual Meeting of the British Paediatric Association in 1990.[70] The short-term outcome was greatly influenced by the multiple adverse family factors, educational and social factors amongst these families [Table 19]. Prospective research was clearly required to clarify all the factors that determine the long-term outcome and the best interests of these children.

Newborn babies 'at risk'

A noteworthy part of the work at the Family Unit, as at the Mother and Child Unit at the Fleming Hospital, was the assessment and support of families with newborn babies at severe risk of harm and neglect at the hands of their parents or caretakers. These were families with serious dysfunctions, often with limited abilities, chaotic lifestyles and social deprivation. Many had harmed or neglected other children before, but in others it concerned the mother's first child.

During a 16-year period from 1978 to 1993, 164 newborn babies were admitted with their mothers and eventually with some of their fathers for a family assessment [Tables 20, 21, 22]. This was a significant experience in a most sensitive and difficult area of child care. The removal of a baby from the mother and family at or soon after birth is one of the most draconian and distressing actions for parents and all concerned. At that time in Newcastle and the northern districts, the alternative to a residential assessment would have been immediate reception into care in many of these cases, with all the practical difficulties of making assessments of bonding and quality of care during the early weeks of life under these circumstances. There was one other residential facility in the city that catered specifically for these problems and undertook family assessments; the Ryehill Family Care Centre under the aegis of the Social Services Department.[71a] Following the initial assessment, this centre could continue to support and help families for a much longer period of several months or more. These activities in the health as well as the social services were strongly supported by Mr Brian Roycroft, the first Director of the Newcastle Social Services Department created in 1971. He worked closely with Dr Cooper and

75

was also President of the Association of Directors of Social Services. He has been described following his death in 2002, as "one of the most charismatic and influential social services director of the last 30 years."[71b]

The facilities of the Mother and Child Unit at the Fleming Memorial Hospital and the Family Unit at Newcastle General Hospital were not suited for long term purposes, but provided an additional element in the network of services for these families.

There was considerable interest and concern about these problems in the 1970s and early 1980s. An important study was published in 1980 about 160 babies taken into statutory care in Britain at or soon after birth in the previous seven years. The title of the article "Removing Babies at birth. A questionable practice" expressed the substantial concerns about the measures adopted during that era to protect these babies.[72] It was written by a consultant child psychiatrist and an area social services officer. The total number was thought to represent a considerable under-estimate. Child abuse or neglect had occurred in most (76%), and statutory action was also reported for 16 first-born babies. Significantly, unlike the experience at the Newcastle Units, major psychiatric factors including schizophrenia and severe mental disability were reported in half the cases. It was noted:

"The practice was more widespread than was generally imagined, with doctors and nurses always concerned."

And it was recommended:

"More detailed surveillance of statutory care actions at birth and in the first three months of life be undertaken."

Lawyers were also concerned about a "pre-emptive strike" and even wrote emotively about "the legal implications of this form of baby-snatching."[73]

Dr Cooper had already written in 1979[74] and taught:

"Removal of the baby from his mother damages her capacity to care for him. Parents already vulnerable to difficulties thus have their problems with the baby magnified."

She went on to give an account of her views, which inspired her teaching and the clinical work, which she initiated at the Babies Hospital. It is one of the most lucid and comprehensive accounts of the issues that need to be considered:

"Unless we are certain that the parents can never care for the child, we must do all we can to keep mother and baby together for a while. If necessary, this must be done under legal controls so that a proper assessment of the family can be made. In such cases a full psychological study of the parents and family is needed. This must include the parents' hopes and feelings about the newborn

76

baby; their personal biographies; the social situation; and their relationship to each other, to their other children, to the extended family, and to neighbours and friends. Each child born may give parents new hope and a new start; when the spouse has changed, material conditions are better, or time and professional help have brought some improved understanding and maturity, it is possible that they can care for this child safely when they could not cope with others. Events around the birth and the first days of life may also influence the picture."

By the 1980s, there was an expectation by the courts in Newcastle and the northern region that a thorough residential assessment of the family should be done about the quality of attachment and care of the newborn baby before a recommendation about future care is made. This was in part due to Dr Cooper's pioneering work.

The resources, ambience and experience at the Family Unit were suited for this purpose and a relatively short time in residence in a safe environment for a period of six to eight weeks was usually considered to be sufficient in this age group to complete an assessment and make recommendations at the concluding multi-disciplinary case conference. Support and help would then continue at home.

Even when babies were taken away from their parents after a few weeks, it was evident that some of them, having had the opportunity to know and care for their child, were better able to mourn their loss. The staff of the Family Unit, who had come to know the parents and were almost always able to engage with them, were in a position to support them at such a distressing conclusion. It was felt that avoidable harm is done to parents by removing a baby at birth or soon after in the belief of protecting them from further distress. The safety of the baby could be ensured in the environment of the hospital facilities.

Two separate reviews were undertaken in relation to newborn babies 'at risk' admitted to the FMH and NGH. There is an overlap of 12 cases in 1989. The first review from 1978 to 1989 was concerned primarily with outcome, the second from 1989 to 1993 with the additional processes of assessment and consideration of antecedent risk factors. This accounts for the differences in the data [Table 20].

A significant proportion of newborn babies were taken into care after the residential assessments. It increased from 19% to 30% during the later years. This was a reflection of the increasing complexities and high risks of the referrals as the reputation of the Family Unit became established. The attempts to ensure the protection of the first born were a particular challenge. They represented half of the newborns 'at risk' during 1978-1989 and rather fewer (36%) during 1989-1993 as community services were developing to cater for these problems.

Information about longer term outcome in those assessed during the first period of 1978-1989 is limited to the first 12-18 months only after the end of the residential assessment. Out of 115, 81% were discharged home but 19% of these were later taken into foster care, leaving only 64.5% still at home 12-18 months later. Amongst the 58 first born, 66% were still at home with rather fewer (60%) amongst the 53 with a history of at least one previous child taken into care. These findings were presented to the community paediatrics group at the annual meeting of the British Paediatric Association in 1990.[75]

An analysis of the short-term outcome during 1978 to 1987 revealed an unfavourable outcome in the high proportion of families with learning difficulties (42%), very young mothers, and when there had been abuse, neglect or inability to care for previous children [Table 21]. Families with both parents with learning difficulties fared the worst; nearly three-quarters of their newborn babies went into foster care. Overall, only 40 (56%) out of 72 were allowed home after the assessment at the Family Unit. In the second survey from 1989 to 1993 [Table 22], there is no separate identification of parents with learning difficulties. As in previous years, concerns about past abuse, neglect and safe care figure prominently. At least one previous child had been taken into care in over half of the families and a third had more than two previous children removed from their care. The information about the 22 first born babies gives an indication of the high risk factors that prompted the assessment of their families. There was a history of violence by the father in about a third and concerns about the ability of the mother to provide appropriate and safe care in the remainder. There was thus a great deal of concern about safety and a realisation that the problems of these families during this five-year period were ever more challenging. Overall, there was a decrease in the proportion of babies discharged home on the completion of the assessments - 70% compared with 81% - during the previous decade. A further indication of increasing difficulties was the large proportion of assessments that had to be terminated before completion – 10 out of the 18 taken into foster care – because of the disruptive behaviour of the parents and caretakers at the Family Unit or their inability and unwillingness to complete the assessments.

A case history illustrates the sophistication of the assessments undertaken by 1995 and the considerable resources deployed to try to ensure the welfare and safety of the child.[76]

Baby 'Michael' and his parents were referred to the Family Unit by a consultant paediatrician on the recommendation of a child protection case conference. There was concern for his safety as two older siblings, a four year old and a two year old were the subject of Care Orders and awaiting adoption. At the age of 10 weeks, the younger child had been admitted to hospital with gastro-enteritis and was also noted to have bruising to her face, which was about 3 days old. There was also a history of bruising to her eyes at the age of 3 weeks. A skeletal survey revealed three fractured ribs and a healing fracture of the femur. A diagnosis of non-accidental injuries was made. The oldest child, at that time, had no injuries apart from a few small bruises and scratches consistent with the explanation of the parents. Both children were placed with foster parents. The father admitted injuring the baby and received a 12 months custodial sentence. Although their relationship was erratic, the parents remained together and baby 'Michael' was conceived. During the mother's pregnancy, the social services asked the NSPCC to undertake a formal risk assessment before the baby's birth. This identified three key areas that needed to be addressed with the parents:

The need to understand how the injuries to their previous child had occurred.
The need to find out what had changed for the parents since the time of the injury.
More needed to be done to find out about the nature and quality of the relationship between the parents both currently and at the time of injuries.

It was arranged for the mother with her new baby to remain in the maternity hospital for two weeks and then for the mother and the baby to live with foster parents. The father was allowed two hours a day supervised contact with his baby at the local Family Centre and an Interim Care Order under the Children's Act of 1989 was obtained. Seven weeks after his birth, a place became available at the Family Unit. The assessment was based on nursing observations and psychological and psychiatric assessments. The unit's overall assessment demonstrated the parent's positive attachment to the child, a recognition of their past failures as parents, an ability to respond to professional advice, an appreciation of the need for continuing support and monitoring of their roles as parents and their willingness to cooperate with professionals. The clinical psychologist's assessment of the mother revealed that she had below average verbal-cognitive abilities, poor self-confidence and very high dependency needs for emotional support and guidance to cope with her feelings of insecurity and vulnerability. The father's verbal-cognitive abilities were also below average and his style of communication suggested poor underlying self-confidence, further highlighted by a tendency to bottle up or avoid talking about his feelings. The psychiatric assessment of both parents was carried out by a consultant in Child and Adolescent Psychiatry. These assessments were concerned with the events surrounding the injuries and the changes that had taken place in the family since these events.
A case conference with the parents, social workers, NSPCC, Community Family Centre workers, health visitors, members of the Family Unit assessment team and the guardian ad litem recommended that the child should return home to the parents.
Assessment in the community by the NSPCC would continue. The application for a full Care Order by the Social Services would also continue with the possibility of a change to a Supervision Order if things went well when the case went back to court. The parents and baby were discharged home a week later when a comprehensive package of support and supervision in the community had been organised. The baby was healthy and was thriving under their care.

Comment
This case history illustrates the considerable resources that had to be deployed in order to try to safeguard the health and welfare of this child. These parents with limited abilities and personal emotional resources would need prolonged community support. The Family Unit played a central part in arriving at a recommendation to allow the baby home as part of an extensive network of

expert services in close collaboration with each other. The contributions of Child Psychology and Psychiatry to the assessments were of critical importance.

The favourable outcome for the family, at least in the short term, is a vindication of Dr Cooper's insight and teaching that parents might be helped and able to care for their new baby, even under the cloud of severe physical abuse in the past. Also that effective expert services were needed on a long-term basis in order to guide and support them. The NSPCC's involvement is of great interest. It was always very active in Newcastle and the north east of England long before the second half of the 20th century.

It was evident in these cases as in all the categories of abuse and neglect presenting at the Family Unit, that long term prospective follow-up studies were required in order to determine the safest and best way to protect these children and treat and support their families.

After 1989 there was a significant change in the law, which eventually had an important impact on the safeguard of newborns 'at risk' and the process of assessment and care for all children from 'vulnerable' families. It involved:

"A change in philosophy, moving from the concept of parental rights towards the rights of the child, whilst emphasising cooperation and the sharing of parental responsibilities."[77]

A further important change was that the court "shall not make an order unless it considers that doing so would be better for the child than making no order at all." This was to discourage unnecessary protection orders.[78] The intention was to reduce conflict and promote parental agreement and cooperation.

As a result, by the time the Act was fully implemented in 1991 no further Wardship Orders and few Care Orders were sought by Social Services before the admission of newborn babies 'at risk' to the Family Unit. Compared with the three years before 1991 when 30 (86%) out of 35 were on legal orders on admission for a family assessment, only three (11.5%) out of 26 were admitted on Interim Care Orders in the two years after 1991 [Table 22].

The same applied to older infants who had been abused and neglected. This put a considerable onus on the community social and health services to provide safe environments and effective assessment of 'vulnerable' families. The same applied to the Family Unit during those years to ensure the safety of the child without the added support of legal controls in most cases. A further understanding of legal considerations had to be included in paediatric practice.

Child Sexual Abuse (CSA)

CSA was suddenly identified as a significant priority for paediatrics in Newcastle and the northern region during the middle of the 1980s. The same applied to the rest of the country. New skills and attitudes had to be learnt rapidly by paediatricians. A knowledge and experience of family, social and environmental factors affecting childhood also had to be deployed in order to participate effectively in the complex multidisciplinary activities that were

80

required for the diagnosis and further management of these children and their families.

Only a very small number of children with CSA were ever admitted for a residential assessment. They are included in this study because historically they represent a watershed in the greater understanding of the nature and extent of the problem in the community. Dr Cooper was well aware of the condition and dealt with some cases. She did not make use of the residential hospital facilities for this purpose. In 1987 shortly before the closure of the Mother and Child Unit at the FMH, three children from two families were admitted for a second opinion of a CSA diagnosis made by a consultant paediatrician in Cleveland. They were part of a group of 49 children under the age of 5 years amongst the 120 diagnosed over a relatively short period of three months at Middlesbrough General Hospital. This was an unprecedented number over such a short period of time and caused a great deal of consternation about the security of the diagnosis and the method of further management, as a majority were admitted to the paediatric wards on Place of Safety Orders.[79] One of the three children went back home from the FMH to the care of her mother, with the father asked to leave home while enquiries were proceeding. He was eventually allowed home on the order of the court. The other two from the same family went into foster care for several months until they were readmitted to the Family Unit at NGH with both parents for a joint assessment of the family with child psychology and psychiatry. They were by then Wards of Court, did well and were allowed home on discharge from the unit. A year later, the family was settled and the children were progressing normally.

There was a crisis in the northern region, which had an impact on the Family Unit and further afield as it alerted paediatricians for the first time to the complex nature of the presentation and the wide extent of the problem. Social services were well aware of the situation – in 1986, the NSPCC had recorded 527 children with suspected CSA on their register, an incidence of 0.57 per 1000 children aged 16 or less.[79] Also in the northern region, a scheme to provide female forensic examiners for the police in cases of suspected sexual assault had been set up in 1983.[80] The Northumbria Women Police Doctors consisted of general practitioners, community child health doctors, a number of junior hospital paediatricians, a consultant paediatrician, Dr Margaret Taylor of South Shields Hospital and later, Dr Camille Lazaro, senior registrar in paediatrics at the RVI. There was thus already a pool of expertise in the community, but aside from the few paediatricians involved, experience in paediatrics generally was severely limited. This was a significant disadvantage particularly as potential victims amongst young children were increasingly identified by social services. Most consultant paediatricians during that era had little or no knowledge and experience in the identification, care and management of these children and their families.

A Judicial Inquiry was set up by the contemporary Secretary of State, John Moore, MP and a report was presented to Parliament in July 1988. It was led by Lord Justice Butler-Sloss.[81] Dr Liam Donaldson, the northern regional medical officer (later Professor Sir Liam and chief medical officer for England) convened two Second Opinion Panels in order to assist the Inquiry and 'calm'

81

the situation. Professor Kolvin from the Nuffield Child Psychiatry Unit in Newcastle chaired the Panels, which consisted of consultant paediatricians and child psychiatrists from Tyneside and further afield, (Manchester, Leeds, Oxford and London). Assessments were undertaken jointly between the paediatricians and child psychiatrists in the children and members families referred by the Cleveland Social Services Department and under review by the Judicial Inquiry.

The other Panel consisted of consultant paediatricians from Newcastle and surrounding districts, who were to be called to provide a second opinion on children referred to Cleveland paediatricians during the course of the Inquiry, with suspected sexual abuse. Police surgeons, who had assessed some of these children, also took part and some were present during the assessments by the paediatricians. These were temporary arrangements during the course of the Inquiry. They were intended to assist the paediatricians in Cleveland and provide additional 'reassurance' to the public at a time of considerable upheaval and controversy.

H.S. from the Family Unit was invited to join the panels. A report was presented to the inquiry. It recommended a multidisciplinary approach to diagnosis and a response commensurate with the likelihood of CSA having taken place.[82] A special feature of the panels' assessments involved a joint paediatric and child psychiatry opinion. This was precisely the mechanism that had evolved at the Mother and Child Unit at the FMH and the Family Unit at NGH. It demonstrated the potential value of such an arrangement.

For some months in 1988, a few children under the age of 5 years with suspected CSA were referred as outpatients by social services and seen with their mother and social worker at the Family Unit. Ten children were examined for evidence of CSA, ill health, adverse growth and development and evidence of abnormal behaviour. All were entirely normal and the home circumstances appeared to be satisfactory. All went home to be followed up by the primary health care and social services. The police were still investigating some of the circumstances.

This was a time during which there was a steep learning curve to cope with these problems. The experience was similar to that of many paediatricians nationwide.

A review of the literature about the physical signs of child sexual abuse was undertaken, resulting in a joint publication by H.S and Dr Margaret Taylor, who had considerable experience of the diagnosis as a result of her work over many years at the request of the police and social services in South Shields. A precise, standard examination and consistent recording were described.[83]

These experiences led to a review of the records of a sample of families with issues of child protection, looking for any indications of a history of sexual abuse early in the life of the parents. This had not been routinely sought, but emerged in social services records and the notes of the residential assessments. By that time, it was no surprise to find that a significant proportion of mothers had been abused [Table 23]. The number of mothers affected was almost certainly an underestimate. These insights were incorporated in later family assessments.

No further arrangements were made to see children with suspected CSA at the Family Unit as a comprehensive regional service was set up by Dr Camille Lazaro at the Lindisfarne Centre in the Children Clinic at the RVI. She was appointed Senior Lecturer in Paediatric Forensic Medicine and consultant paediatrician in late 1989 in order to cater for children in Newcastle and the northern region, train doctors and health service staff and undertake research. An indication of the significant extent of suspected CSA in the childhood population of the northern region is the large number of children referred very quickly to this new service every year.[84] By 2001-2, there were over 600 new referrals amongst a total of over 900 children attending the centre during those years, with some coming as far afield as the Isle of Man.[85] Dr Lazaro was awarded the OBE for her services to these children and their families. At the same time, the Family Unit at NGH was still available to participate in the multidisciplinary assessment of the families, especially those with young children taken into foster care after an initial diagnosis of CSA.

The changes and closure of the Family Unit, 1995-1997

A significant change took place at the Family Unit following the retirement at the end of 1994 of the consultant paediatrician responsible for the clinical work of the Family Unit. H.S. had followed in the footsteps of Dr Cooper since 1983 and was, as in her case, the only consultant paediatrician undertaking this kind of work in a specialist hospital facility in Newcastle and the northern region. Most of the other consultant paediatricians in the city and the region were involved in the initial clinical diagnosis of non-accidental injuries and neglect during the later decades of the 20th century. They were not directly concerned with the subsequent family assessments and multidisciplinary measures that are needed to determine the fate of the children thereafter. No other consultant paediatrician was available and ready to take on this work at the Family Unit. As a result, responsibility was taken over by the staff of the Nuffield Child Psychology and Psychiatry Department of Newcastle, who were already participating in the assessments. The service continued as before but with a diminishing number of referrals as community services took over.[86]

The Family Unit eventually closed in 1997 two decades after the beginning of the service at the Fleming Hospital for vulnerable families who had abused or neglected their children or were at risk of doing so. The resources required for a residential hospital assessment and support of these families could no longer be sustained. The National Health Service could not continue to finance the service and the Social Services were unable to do so. The consultant psychologist and child psychiatrists were also restricted to some extent by the lack of active involvement with paediatricians and the practical difficulties of maintaining control of the increasing disruptive behaviour of some parents and caretakers within the confines of a hospital setting. The nursing staff and nursery nurse also had increasing anxieties about the safety of the children under these circumstances.[86] The high rate of breakdowns of the assessments of families with newborn babies 'at risk' already noted in 1989-1993 [Table 22] illustrates some of the difficulties that were encountered.

The admission of severely disabled children for respite care ended in 1996 as provisions increased elsewhere.

Only a handful of rooms had ever been available to undertake this work with vulnerable families after the closure of the Babies Hospital at Leazes Terrace in 1976. There were seven at the Mother and Child Unit at the Fleming Hospital in 1977 to 1987 and five at the Family Unit during 1988 to 1991 [Table 13], with a similar number during the final six years of that Unit. The average length of stay of the families was relatively short, 3-4 weeks at the Fleming Memorial Hospital [Table 14a] and 6-8 weeks at Newcastle General Hospital [Table 17]. During a 14 year period from March 1977 to April 1991, 650 children were admitted from families with "psycho-social problems" during that era.[14] In 1991, it was still the custom to refer to the problems of these families as "psycho-social' in nature. This was in keeping with the combination of psychological and social problems that were being identified and in recognition of the contribution of psychology and psychiatry to the assessments. Later, 'child protection' came into common usage, reflecting a change in outlook and the increasing sophistication of the multidisciplinary activities that were developing. These were young children under the age of 3 years and a majority under the age of 1 year. The risks of harm to these children varied. Some of the families required only additional support, help and supervision at home. In others there were significant child protection issues that required statutory action to secure the welfare and safety of the children in substitute families.

In 1996 a few months before the closure of the Family Unit, a survey was undertaken to determine the outcome in families who had an assessment there during two years from 1992 to 1994. Information was gathered by Sister Greenacre, the nursery nurse Christine Cardose and the nursing staff. The consultant psychologist, Dr Trian Fundudis and the consultant child psychiatrists, Dr Carole Kaplan, Dr Paul McArdle and Dr Sue Wressel from the Nuffield Child Psychiatry Unit were closely involved. The 'key' social worker or the health visitor when appropriate were contacted by telephone and data collected with the help of a questionnaire [Tables C and 26-31].[87]

This was the most complete of all the surveys of outcome in families admitted for an assessment for purposes of child protection during the period of 15 years from 1979 to 1994. Information was obtained in all but one of the 69 families assessed during 1992 to 1994. Eighty children were involved. Most of them were very young with just over half less than 6 months old and 75% under the age of 1 year, so that by the time of their follow up in July-August 1996, the majority were 3-5 years old and only seven were less than 2 years of age.

These 68 families had many problems: nearly half were single parents. Case histories indicate that nearly all had multiple family and social problems. They were already well known to social services and had received a great deal of help and support in the past. Strikingly, in the 26 families with previous children, all these children were in the care of local authorities or other family members.

A majority (62.5%) was allowed to go home to the care of their parents after the residential assessment. One child went to live with another family

84

member (the grandmother). However, less than half (46%) of the children were still with their parents or caretakers two to four years later.

Very few Care Orders were sought and there were no more Wardship Orders. This was in keeping with the provisions of the 1989 Children Act, which emphasised parental responsibility and limitation of legal orders if the child was in a safe environment and the parents were cooperating with the help and support that was offered to them.

An attempt to rehabilitate children to the care of their parents continued after discharge from the Family Unit in a significant proportion of the children not allowed to go home after the assessment. Three were discharged to another residential establishment able to cater for families on a long-term basis; none of these families completed this further assessment and all these children went to foster parents. Ten children already in foster homes were considered for a return home; only one was successful.

A significant proportion of the mothers (about a third) had further children by 1996. This applied equally to those with children in foster care or adopted as in those with their children at home.

Infants with non-accidental injuries fared the best. A majority of those discharged to the care of their parents and caretakers (62%) were still with them two to four years later. Sadly, one child with a history of a single fracture and bruising, who went home after the residential assessment had a further injury. The severity is not known [Table 29].

The 'dysfunctional' families had the worst outcome. Less than half (45%) were allowed home after the assessment at the Family Unit and less than a third (27%) were still there in 1996 [Table 31].

The majority of the newborn babies at risk (76% of the original 33) were allowed home, but only 45% were still at home at the time of the survey and there had been one cot death [Table 30]. This may have been fortuitous, but there is a well established association with social deprivation and a past history of abuse and neglect.[88]

Some of the families had such worrying problems, which appeared to pose such severe risks to their children, that care in their families would probably not even have been considered if residential assessments had not been available. The contributions of child psychology and psychiatry were especially fruitful.

The six surveys of outcome of families assessed during the 16 years from 1978 to 1994 [Table C] indicate a decline over a period of ten years in successful care of vulnerable children by their parents or caretakers. This can be attributed in the main to a distinct increase in the severity and complexity of the problems of these families, which were referred to the Family Unit.

The limitations of the information during those years of child protection indicate the need for well planned, long-term follow up studies of outcome, which were never achieved.

The birth of so many children after the assessments at the Family Unit, especially in families with children already taken into care, suggests the need for additional support and vigilance on a long-term basis by all the community services. This could provide opportunities to prevent abuse and neglect by helping families to take better care of their children in the future and break the 'cycle of deprivation'.

The reputation of the Family Unit as a valuable resource had grown over the years. The commitment initiated by Dr Cooper to try to help some of the most vulnerable families at greatest risk of harming and neglecting their children and the ready participation of paediatrics in multidisciplinary activities with the community services came to be widely accepted. The development of effective, amicable collaboration between paediatrics, child psychology, child psychiatry and the nursing staff was ultimately the basis for the attempt to participate in the protection of the children and the support that was given to their families during those years by the community services.

Table C Surveys of children admitted to the Mother and Child Unit at the Fleming Memorial Hospital for Sick Children and the Family Unit at Newcastle General Hospital. 1978-1994

	1979 – 89 Family Unit			1978 – 91 Family Unit			1984 – 85 Mother and Child Unit			1988 – 91 (1 April) Family Unit		1989 – 93 Family Unit		1992 – 94 Family Unit		
	Total	Discharged home	At home after 12-18 months	Total	Discharged home	At home after average of 16 months	Total	Discharged home	Still at home in 1986	Total	Discharged home	Total	Discharged home	Total	Discharged with parents [2]	Still at home in 1996
Newborn at risk	115	93 81%	74 64%				25	21 84%	17 68%	43		61	43 70%	33	25 76%	15 [3] 45%
Non-accidental injuries				26	17 65%	15 58%	16	10 63%	10 63%	26 [1]				21	14 67%	13 62%
Problems of care. Dysfunctional families							16	13 81%	12 75%	37				23	10 45%	6 27%
Unharmed siblings							7	5	7	-				4	4	4
Total number of children							64	49 77%	44 69%	117	81 69%			80	50 [4] 62.5%	37 46%

Notes:

1. Includes five who were sexually abused
2. Three others discharged to a longer-term residential establishment with their parents for a further assessment with a view to rehabilitation (None were eventually rehabilitated)
3. One child died at home – cot death.
4. One other child was discharged to the care of grandparents after the original assessment

It is a matter of great regret that it was not possible to undertake prospective follow up studies on a long-term basis. The considerable resources required to do so were simply not available.

There is no recorded data for the last three years of the Family Unit. The recollections of the staff and doctors involved indicate that there were only 25 to 30 admissions each year and that the problems of the families had continued to increase. In any case, the need for such a residential hospital assessment had diminished as expertise had been increasing in the community services.[89, 90, 91] The number of referrals to the Family Unit had also been decreasing for several years.

Family centres were set up in the 1970s and ten years later there were 500 nationwide. They were managed by statutory social services departments, consortia or partnerships of self-help, voluntary organisations and other statutory bodies.[61] In Newcastle during the 1980s, the Riverside Child Health Project was providing a community service in the west end of the city where the West End Day Nursery had been established in 1918. A team of paediatricians, social workers and community care workers engaged with local people, primary health care services, hospitals, social services, schools and voluntary associations to help and support the families in that area. Child protection was an important part of their work and the active participation of the families was a fundamental element of the service.[92, 93]

The Family Resource Team of the Newcastle Social Services Department is another example of these new community services. It was set up in 1993 following the closure due to financial constraints of the Ryehill Residential Family Care Centre in the west of the city, which had catered for vulnerable 'problem families' on a long-term basis. The purpose was to provide a community based child protection assessment by social workers and family workers. After 18 months, plans were made to include joint work with child minders and home care workers.[94]

In addition, consultant community paediatricians were by then available to participate in child protection. The value and possible roles of this new branch of paediatrics were studied in Newcastle during the 1970s with promising results[68] and commended in 1976 by the Committee on Child Health Services, chaired by Professor Court.[95] Twenty-six years later in 2002, The Royal College of Paediatrics and Child Health concluded in a review of community child health services:

"The distinction between hospital and community paediatricians had become increasingly artificial and should be phased out."

Patterns of morbidity and care were changing and it was recommended that all paediatricians should have "generic training to be able to cope with the "local" needs of children in acute and chronic paediatrics and child health." Sub-specialisation would inevitably occur and this would include participation in child protection in the community.[96]

Case Histories 1987 - 1991

The Family Unit at Newcastle General Hospital.
Transcribed from the Reports of the Family Unit
at Newcastle General Hospital.[14]

A. Newborn baby with mother — 7 previous children in Care. Abuse and neglect.
Discharged home

B. Newborn baby with mother and father — Past abuse. Multiple fractures.
Discharged home

C. 3 months old baby with mother and father — First child killed by father.
Discharged home

D. Newborn baby with mother — First child of parents with severe learning difficulties.
To foster care

E. 4 months old baby with mother and father — Physical abuse.
Discharged home

F. 1 year old infant with mother and father — Physical abuse.
To foster care

G. 16 months old infant with mother — Failure to thrive and emotional abuse.
To foster care

H. Newborn baby with mother and father — Conviction of father for abuse of unrelated child.
Physical abuse of child (in Care) and later child also in Care.
Discharged home

I. Newborn baby with mother and father — Conviction of father for sexual abuse of young children.
To foster care

J. 2 and a half year old toddler — Sexual abuse of mother in childhood.
To foster care

K. Newborn baby with mother and father — Two previous children in Care.
Physical abuse.
Discharged home

89

Family A. Mother and her newborn baby

The mother was 36 years old and her first seven children were taken into Care. The eldest is now 19 years old. There were varying combinations of neglect, physical abuse and very poor parenting and general care; some of the children had been received into Voluntary Care because mother was unable to cope. She had a most unhappy childhood with periods in foster care and as an adult had numerous unstable relationships with men who were generally violent, abused alcohol and had criminal records. The children were by a variety of different partners. She herself had a history of alcohol abuse, poor self-care, a petty criminal record and a most unstable lifestyle over many years. There had been a considerable amount of social work support over a very long period of time, but the mother had been unable to respond and at times cooperation was very poor. Of particular concern was mother's inability to accept responsibility for failing to look after her children adequately.

Her eighth child was made a Ward of Court and referred for a family assessment by Social Services following a Case Conference recommendation. Mother and baby were transferred from the local maternity unit. During a residential period of 7 weeks it was possible to establish that there was a strong attachment between mother and child, that she was well able to care for him and that she was beginning to develop an increasing awareness of her previous problems and deficiencies. There was also the beginning of an acknowledgement of some responsibility for past events. She was able to respond to support and care, took advice appropriately and made friends with other resident families and the staff of the Unit. Her personal circumstances had changed within her home environment; she was now single and had a good home of her own; she felt that she had 'matured' and that she would not make the mistakes of the past. The baby was well and normal.

A multidisciplinary Case Conference recommended that an attempt be made to help her to look after her child at home.

The family is doing well one year later.

Comment

To date there appears to be a successful outcome. This baby would have been taken into Care soon after birth if the residential facilities at the Family Unit had not been available and it is likely that permission to place the baby in a permanent substitute family would have been sought in the High Court.

Family B. Mother and father and their newborn baby

The first child of this family had been taken into Care at the age of 6 weeks two and a half years before the birth of their second baby. This followed a diagnosis of serious and life threatening non-accidental injuries, which included multiple fractures. Father admitted responsibility. Rehabilitation however did not take place and the baby is now adopted. There were major concerns about the future of the second child.

Unlike many families in which abuse had taken place, there did not appear to be the multiplicity of adverse family, educational, social and environmental factors in the backgrounds of the parents that might predispose to a significant vulnerability and potential for abuse of their children. They were however quite young (mother 18 and father 19) when their first child was born and immature and inexperienced. Father was very possessive towards their first baby, insisting on taking the main burden of care on his shoulders. At the time, he had a low tolerance to stress and became angry when the baby began to cry and be unsettled. Mother was quite unaware of her husband's feelings towards the baby and indeed the impropriety of his violent behaviour towards her. He was prosecuted and given a three year Probation Order, which had recently expired.

The new baby was a Ward of Court and transferred to the Family Unit from the maternity hospital. During a period of seven weeks of assessment, no problems of any kind were encountered. There were strong attachments and the parents were well able to look after their child. Their relationship was loving and stable and they had a good home. There was very good cooperation with the assessment. The baby remained well and was making normal progress.

A Case Conference recommended that the child go home to their care and 2 years later they are still doing well.

Comment in retrospect (2014)

This was one of several families of young parents who had "grown up" and were thereby able take care of their new baby safely and appropriately, despite the damaging past history of serious abuse – a vindication of the teaching of Dr Cooper that each vulnerable family, however worrying their past experiences may have been, should be given the opportunity to try and take care of their new child, because significant improvements in their personal development and social circumstances may have taken place.

The safe and nurturing environment of the Family Unit provided them with a 'haven' that helped them to make a good start and do well.

Family C. Mother and father and their 3 months old baby

Mother's first husband was convicted of the manslaughter of their first child. This had been a particularly brutal physical attack and mother had failed to protect him, failed to get early medical help and indeed failed to alert anyone about the events; she colluded with him in hiding the true facts. She was prosecuted, found guilty, and given a 12 months custodial sentence for wilful neglect. There were thus two years later, major concerns about the welfare of her second child by another partner.

The mother's past history indicates that she had a most unhappy and deprived childhood, lacking in affection with poor examples of parenting. Her father died in an accident when she was 9 years old and her mother subsequently started to drink heavily. She thereafter had to look after herself and also cope with her mother. From the age of about 16 years, she had a number of unstable adult relationships, including marriage to the father of her first child. The man had shown great violence towards her. She herself had a history of excessive drinking and she had left her first child in the care of others when she went out with her mother and was at times too drunk to look after him effectively. This had led to a number of receptions into Voluntary Care before the first assault on the child.

The baby's father also had a most unhappy, deprived and affectionless childhood in a family with many problems. His father had also died when he was young and his mother then began to drink. He was subsequently taken into foster care. In adolescence and adulthood there is a long history of criminal offences leading to custodial sentences. He has two children now aged 4 and 5 years from a previous relationship, but he is no longer in contact with them. There is no history of abuse towards them. He also drank excessively from time to time.

The couple had known each other for about 18 months following his release from prison and their relationship had been unstable for a while, but in recent times they had settled down in their own home, which was described as clean, well kept with good material standards.

Mother had cooperated well in the antenatal period. The baby was made a Ward of Court and went into foster care before a transfer to the Family Unit for a family assessment could be arranged.

This went very well and during the 7 weeks of residence, the parents appeared to have a reasonably good relationship with each other and it was noticeable that they did support each other during this most anxious period in their lives. There was very good cooperation and they were able to make friends. There was a good deal of insight by mother about her past difficulties and she talked about her fear of her first husband in contrast to her present partner. The baby was healthy and developing normally.

A multidisciplinary case conference recommended rehabilitation home after a great deal of heart searching.

18 months later the child is doing well and although there has been some instability in the relationship between the parents, they are still together.

Comment

It was clear to all concerned that a family residential assessment was necessary before any recommendation could be made about the future of the child.

Comment in retrospect (2014)

Fifteen to twenty years after this case history and comments were written, a number of further comments spring to mind.

It was just in such a family that Wardship Orders were no longer made after 1989, as the baby remained in a safe place from the time of birth and the parents were cooperating with all the agencies concerned with the welfare of the child.

Although much time and effort were expended in gathering the details of the past history of the parents with all the attendant concerns about the risks of harm to further children, attempts were made to keep an open mind and ultimately it was the daily observations of the behaviour of the family and the progress of the child over a relatively short period of time that determined the recommendations about future care. The psychological and psychiatric evaluations during the residence were a vital component of the process by providing essential insights into the contemporary condition of the family and indications of future prospects about the likely ability and motivation of the parents to provide an appropriate safe and nurturing environment for their children. Looking back there was no formal psychotherapy arranged for the majority of these 'problem families'. The 'therapy' consisted of the provision of a nurturing, supportive environment followed by help, support and supervision by health and community social services. These would need to continue on a long-term basis; the prospect of further children 'at risk' in so many of these families was a further consideration. Provision of specific psychotherapy for such a relatively large number of needy families would likely to have been unrealistic during that era because of the high cost and resource implications.

It was appreciated that a much longer period of follow up was required to determine the true value of the service that was provided. Everyone was acutely aware at the time of the severe risks involved for the well-being and safety of the child.

Family D. Mother and father with their newborn baby

This was the first child of a married couple with very limited intellectual abilities. They both attended an Adult Training Centre. There were considerable concerns about their ability to care for a child in their home and the problems were compounded by the fact that the baby was born prematurely and had a severe congenital heart condition, which was likely to require corrective surgery.

The baby was a Ward of Court and transferred to the Family Unit from the maternity hospital. During a period of 7 weeks, it became abundantly clear that the parents were quite unable to meet her needs adequately because of their limited abilities and the baby did not thrive well when they were looking after her. When the staff of the Unit took over, the baby began to improve.

Notwithstanding the fact that both parents were strongly attached to her and had a good relationship with each other, a Case Conference convened by the Social Services recommended that it would not be in the baby's best interest to return home with them.

She has remained in foster care since then and an application will be made to the High Court to free her for adoption.

Comment

This family illustrates the distressing circumstances surrounding recommendations about the future of newborn babies when parents just simply do not have the ability to look after their child. It only seemed possible to come to firm conclusions about the best interests of the child following a residential assessment. The baby did not ultimately come to any harm and at least the parents have had the opportunity to know their child, to care for her and to subsequently mourn their loss in a more effective manner than would otherwise have been possible if the baby had been removed immediately or soon after birth.

Comment in retrospect (2014)

When these comments were made in 1988, the community services were not as well developed as in later years after the closure of the Family Unit in 1997. The alternative of a readily available residential facility with experienced paediatric staff and the routine involvement of a child psychologist and child psychiatrist were an attractive alternative to a community assessment for some health and social services in Newcastle and the northern region. It was arguably a cost effective system, which was limited to a relatively short period of time. The use of Wardship and Care Orders was considered by some a necessity not just to protect the child but also in order to allow the process to proceed more smoothly with naturally reluctant and sometimes initially resistant parents. Arguably too, the legal oversight of the courts did have a positive influence because it provided extra protection for the rights of parents and in some of the most difficult and contentious cases, reassurance and protection for the professionals responsible for the welfare and safety of the child.

The change of emphasis enshrined in the Children Act of 1989, which expected parents to take responsibility and protection services to work more closely with them, occurred at a time when multidisciplinary community services were developing better forms of assessment and multidisciplinary systems to protect children. At this time also, the NHS and social services could no longer sustain the costs of expensive residential resources, let alone the considerable fees of the legal processes.

The eventual closure of the Family Unit in 1997, the last descendant of the original Babies Hospital, occurred in the climate of these developments.

Family E. Mother and father and 4 month old baby

Non-accidental injuries were diagnosed at the age of 2 months. These included bruises on the front of the chest and healing fractures of the shaft of the left tibia, the left 6th rib and the right 9th rib. These fractures were of different ages and the explanation by the parents that an accident had occurred whilst the baby was sitting on mother's lap in the back of a car that had to make an emergency stop was not accepted. This was partly due to the appearance of the injuries, but most importantly because the injuries appeared older than would have been expected. A place of Safety Order had been obtained but the magistrate court declined to grant the Local Authority's application for a Care Order. Instead, it was agreed that the baby should reside at the home of the paternal grandparents pending further assessment. A multidisciplinary Case Conference subsequently recommended referral of the family to the Family Unit.

The assessment showed that the baby was fit and well, that there was a strong attachment with the parents, who were proud of her and were well able to look after her. The relationship between the parents appeared to be a loving one and they supported each other at a very distressing time. The parents had a stable relationship over a considerable period of time and this was their first child. She had been a planned and much wanted baby and they were delighted with her.

There were considerable feeding difficulties during the first month or so with much crying after feeds and it is clear that the parents were very disturbed and distressed with their inability to cope. These were the only stressful events identified in the past history and both parents appeared to have had a happy childhood and adolescence. Father was in regular employment. The only other feature that came to light was his perception that he had been "ham-fisted" and rather "clumsy" in his handling of the baby, but this was not a feature that was observed during the residential assessment.

No further explanation of the injuries came to light. The parents did however acknowledge the seriousness of these injuries and accepted some responsibility for them in the sense that the child was in their care when they must have occurred. They nevertheless categorically denied that they deliberately caused any harm to her.

Interviews of the extended family confirmed that the baby had been happy, was thriving and that there had been a good relationship between the parents.

A multidisciplinary Case Conference recommended rehabilitation home. Four years later the baby is doing well in the care of her mother. The parents have now separated, but are still on amicable terms.

Comment

This family illustrates the possibility of considering rehabilitation of a child home to the care of parents despite a lack of complete knowledge of the cause of physical injuries. There was no 'confession', but only an acknowledgement of difficulties. Other positive factors that came to light during the residential assessment, together with a consideration of the positive elements of the past history allowed a recommendation to be made for rehabilitation.

Comment in retrospect (2014)

The view that was taken in some cases of non-accidental injuries - especially those associated with fractures in very young children - to recommend rehabilitation despite the absence of a full confession was hugely controversial and was not accepted in some cases by some paediatricians and the courts.

It was felt by some that unacceptable risks were taken. At the time we could find no systematic objective evidence that this was an essential condition for attempting rehabilitation, provided that the outlook from the viewpoint of objective observations of parental care, attachment and good relationships was positive and that parents acknowledged that the injuries must have occurred in their care and in that sense accepted some responsibility. It is a matter of considerable regret that long-term follow up studies were not carried out to determine the eventual fate of these families.

Family F. Mother, father and their 10 month old baby

A diagnosis of non-accidental injuries was made at the age of seven months. These included bruising on the chest and buttock, a torn frenulum and multiple fractures of both femurs, the right humerus, the left ulna, the right tibia and one of the lumbar vertebrae. Some of the bone injuries were of different ages. There was no satisfactory explanation for any of these injuries. There was no evidence of any bone disorder in the baby to explain his injuries. The baby was on a Care Order.

Both parents who were unmarried had unhappy backgrounds. Mother had an unsuccessful marriage at the age of 19 years, which ended in divorce 3 years later. She was socially very isolated. Father's parents divorced when he was 7 years old and he was brought up by his grandmother. He had a history of violent behaviour, which had resulted in Court convictions. Although the parents claimed to have had a stable relationship for many months, they had not actually lived together in the same house.

During the residential assessment it was evident that both parents were attached to their child, but it was noticeable that mother did practically all his basic care and at times positively discouraged the father from taking part. The relationship between the parents was noted to be very tense, with many arguments between them, some of them related to the details of the baby's care. It was also clear that the parents often failed to communicate with each other and complained that this had been a significant feature in their lives together.

Mother also began to talk about her own difficulties in communicating her feelings. They seemed unable to resolve their day to day problems in a rational and amicable way. It was significant at the time that this was the first time that the parents had lived together on a 24 hour basis and the father in particular had found it very inhibiting and difficult. They had no specific plans to make a home together in the event of the child's return home, although they reiterated that they would eventually marry. The child was well and normal.

In the event, it was not possible to recommend rehabilitation home and this was accepted by a multidisciplinary Case Conference.

Comment

The state of the relationship between the parents made it impossible for us to recommend rehabilitation. Although it was already clear to the community services that the relationship was suboptimal, the day to day observations in a residential setting highlighted and confirmed their difficulties.

Comment in retrospect (2014)

This was one of the most extreme cases of inflicted physical injuries on a child admitted to the hospital units for a family assessment. There were only two referrals over the years of children with head injuries. It is not made clear in the commentary written at the time that because the parents showed no acceptance whatsoever or any responsibility for such severe harm to the child, that this played a vital part in the recommendation not to rehabilitate. Recollections of this family are sufficiently vivid to record now that this was the case.

It is also evident in retrospect that a residential assessment did not really contribute materially to the final decision. In later years, a preliminary community based assessment, as for example by the NSPCC as described above in the case history of 'Michael', would have been done. At the time there was often considerable pressure on social services to make use of every available residential means before making the final recommendation of permanent placement into care. This was sometimes emphasised in court proceedings. In

Newcastle, the Family Unit was one of two residential facilities that undertook this work and had acquired a positive reputation throughout the northern region as a useful contribution to the multidisciplinary network of resources for child protection. The other centre was the Newcastle social services' Ryehill Centre in the west of the city, which had the resources for a much longer period of residence for assessment, support and training; the number of families that could be catered for there however was limited, with priority given to Newcastle residents.

Family G. A mother and her 16 month old child

Following the admission of the child to another hospital with a febrile convulsion, there was considerable concern because on recovery she presented a picture of a very deprived child with developmental delay. It was also noted on the children's ward that mother did not relate to her at all well and generally seemed unable to respond to her adequately. There had already been considerable concern in the past because of failure to thrive, which became worse when she was 10 months old following the breakup of her family, when her mother found it necessary to look after her on her own. She went to live in a women's hostel and a great deal of support and help from a social worker, health visitor and psychologist were provided.

The mother had a most unhappy childhood. Her life had been extremely restricted, particularly by her father, who did not allow any friendships outside the home, especially with the opposite sex. He sexually abused her from the age of about 11 years and this had only come to light in recent months. It also transpired that he had similarly abused two of her sisters: he was convicted and is now in prison.

Mother herself had many problems. She had epilepsy, a poor self esteem and there have been considerable periods in the past when she was not eating properly. Her family broke up as a direct result of her revelation of sexual abuse in childhood and it is clear that up to that time, her family had taken a considerable part in the care of her child.

As an adult, she had a number of short lived and unstable relationships and had been unhappy and depressed at times. It was also clear that she had considerable difficulties, not only in caring for her child but also for herself and this included home management and budgeting. Despite a considerable input of help, there had been little improvement.

During a six weeks period of residential assessment, there was marked improvement in her child's wellbeing and it was clear that much of her developmental delay was due to a lack of stimulation and inadequate care. We found that mother was quite unable to care for her effectively. She continued to be in a very depressive mood and her relationship with the child was very poor. She relied a great deal on the staff to provide the child's daily care. Although she acknowledged her difficulties and appeared to have considerable insight, she was quite unable to meet the child's needs, as her own needs were so overwhelming. A formal diagnosis of a psychiatric illness was considered, but not confirmed.

It was not possible to recommend a return home and the child who was a Ward of Court went into foster care. An application has been made to the Court to provide her with a permanent substitute home.

Family H. Mother and father with their newborn baby

The parents were in their middle thirties and notwithstanding a number of potentially adverse factors in their past history, the main concern centred on the father's conviction for indecently assaulting an 11 year old girl approximately 11 years before the birth of this baby. This incident occurred at the time of the breakup of his first marriage and apparently consisted 'only' of fondling of the girl's breasts.

He has a history of a disrupted childhood after the divorce of his parents when he was 11 years old. He was currently in regular employment.

His wife is a lady of limited abilities who attended a special school for children with learning difficulties. They had been together for approximately 10 years and had married a year ago. Their relationship had been stable and happy and there had not been any indication of domestic violence. There was support from their extended families.

This baby, who was healthy and normal, was their fourth child. The first one had died five years ago with a congenital heart condition and before that, there had been concern about her welfare because it was felt that she was making inadequate progress. Support and help had been provided by the Social Services Department since infancy.

The second child was removed from their care about 5 years ago at the age of about 4 years, because of a physical assault on her by her father. This consisted of over chastisement when he hit her with a belt on her legs and back. At the time, she was found to be a very disturbed child and her behaviour, which included inappropriate sexual language, suggested that she had been exposed to adult sexual behaviour. There was no evidence of physical sexual abuse. Their third child was also taken into care as a direct result of the concern relating to the other children. The previous two children are in long term foster care with a view to adoption.

The residential assessment suggested that there was a strong bond between the parents and their baby and that they were well able to look after him. He was a normal, healthy baby. There was a good relationship between the parents. The father acknowledged his responsibility for the indecent assault many years ago and maintained that he was full of remorse and that he had not had any inappropriate feelings towards children since that time. His wife confirmed that they had a normal happy relationship and that their family life was stable. They showed a strong commitment to the care of their child.

The assessment of this family was undertaken in close collaboration with a child psychologist, a child psychiatrist and a consultant psychiatrist experienced in the assessment of young people and adults with a history of sexual abuse.

A multidisciplinary Case Conference recommended that the parents be supported to look after their son at home.

THE BABIES' HOSPITAL AND MOTHERCRAFT CENTRE.
Receipts and Payments for the Year ending 31st March, 1926.

RECEIPTS.	£	s.	d.	PAYMENTS.	£	s.	d.	£	s.	d.
GRANT FROM MINISTRY OF HEALTH ...	625	19	2	BALANCES BROUGHT FROM LAST ACCOUNT, DATED 31ST MARCH, 1925				132	18	4
GRANT FROM NEWCASTLE-UPON-TYNE COR-				SALARIES				423	12	6
PORATION	50	0	0	FURNITURE AND EQUIPMENT				265	5	9
MOTHERS' FEES	211	14	3	REPAIRS AND RENEWALS				73	9	1
SUBSCRIPTIONS AND DONATIONS ...	687	7	9	RENTS, RATES AND TAXES				88	12	4
RENT OF GARAGE	14	4	0	FUEL, LIGHTING AND HEATING ...				162	9	6
CO-OPERATIVE SOCIETY DIVIDEND ...	13	10	0	CLEANING AND LAUNDRY				99	3	6
SALE OF UNIFORM MATERIAL ...	7	4	5	FOOD				448	18	2
SALE OF FURNITURE...	4	8	2	CHEMIST				64	4	5
JUMBLE SALES AND ENTERTAINMENTS ...	16	1	3	PRINTING, STATIONERY, ETC. ...				62	2	0
PART PROCEEDS OF BALL	250	0	0	TRAVELLING				14	8	9
PROBATIONERS' FEES	18	1	0	INSURANCE				4	11	4
SUNDRY RECEIPTS	4	16	7	BANK INTEREST AND CHARGES ...				14	0	6
				SUNDRY EXPENSES				3	13	0
				CASH BALANCES—						
				Deposit Account ...	£358	1	0			
				Less—Overdraft on Current Account ...	315	12	1			
					42	8	11			
				Petty Cash in hands of Matron	3	8	6			
								45	17	5
	£1,903	6	7					£1,903	6	7

Audited and Certified Correct
(Signed) SISSON & ALLDEN,
HON. AUDITORS.

NEWCASTLE-UPON-TYNE
16TH JUNE, 1926.

Figure 16: The finances from the First Annual Report. 1925-1926

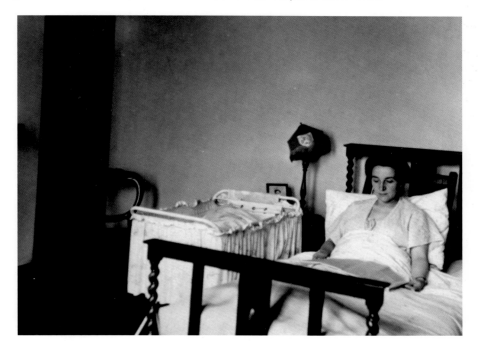

Figure 17: The Princess Mary Maternity Hospital. 1948
Baby's cot at the mother's bedside
Photography Department. King's College, Newcastle

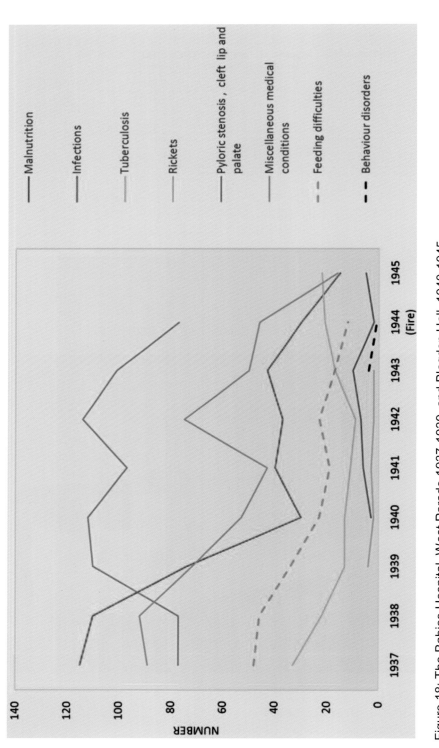

Figure 18: The Babies Hospital, West Parade 1937-1939, and Blagdon Hall. 1940-1945
The changing pattern of diagnoses

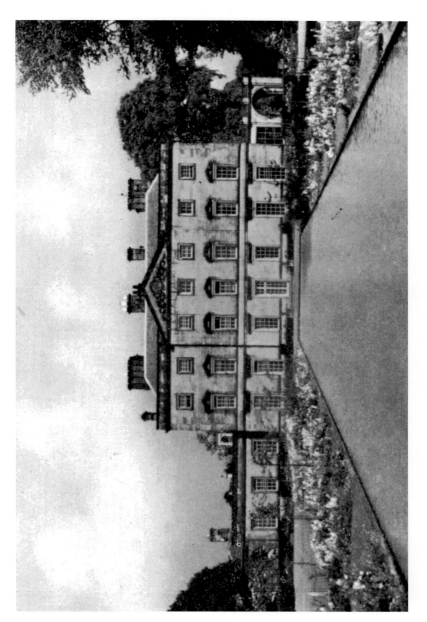

Figure 19: The Babies Hospital at Blagdon Hall, Northumberland 1939 – 1945
Annual Report 1940

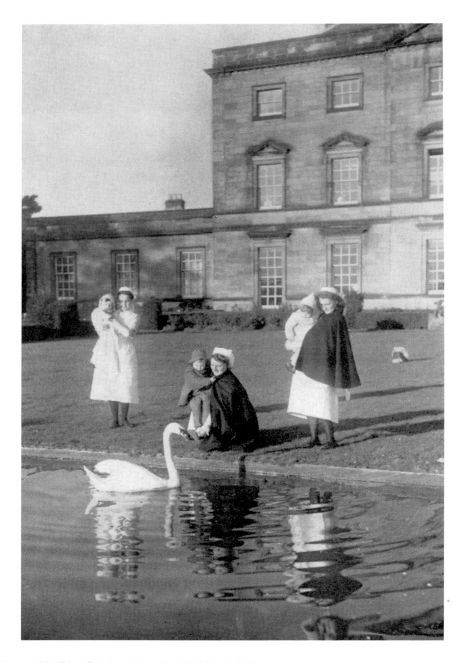

Figure 20: The Babies Hospital 1939 – 1945
Nurses and patients in the garden at Blagdon Hall
Lady Ridley's Memoir.1956

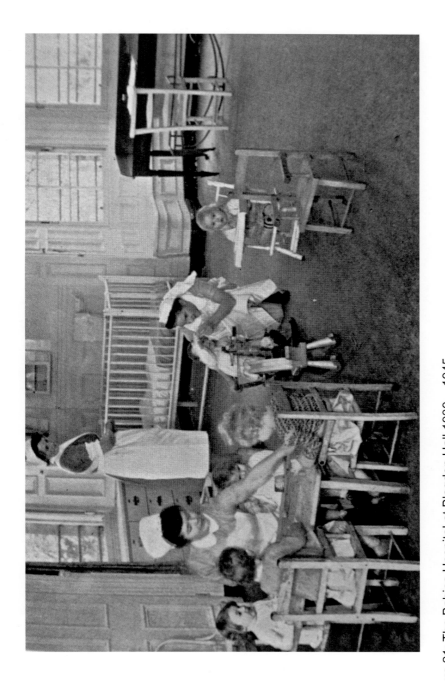

Figure 21: The Babies Hospital at Blagdon Hall 1939 – 1945
Nursery for long stay patients
Lady Ridley's Memoir. 1956

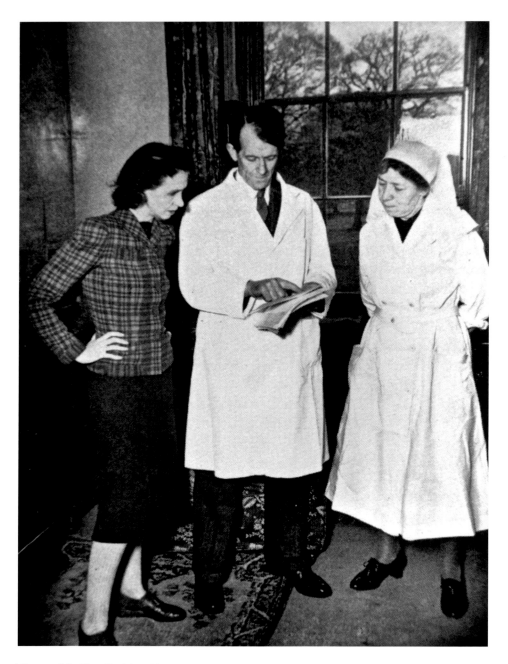

Figure 22: The Babies Hospital
Lady Ridley, Dr Spence and Miss Cummings, who was the matron from 1929 to 1942
Lady Ridley's Memoir. 1956

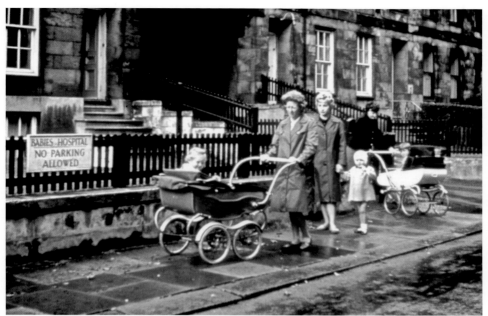

Figure 23a: The Babies Hospital at Leazes Terrace 1966
The Terrace houses at Leazes Terrace

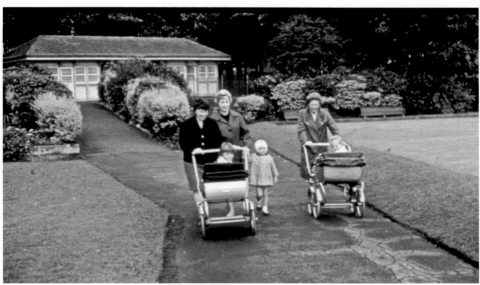

Figure 23b: The Park across the road from Leazes Terrace
Audio Visual Centre. Newcastle University

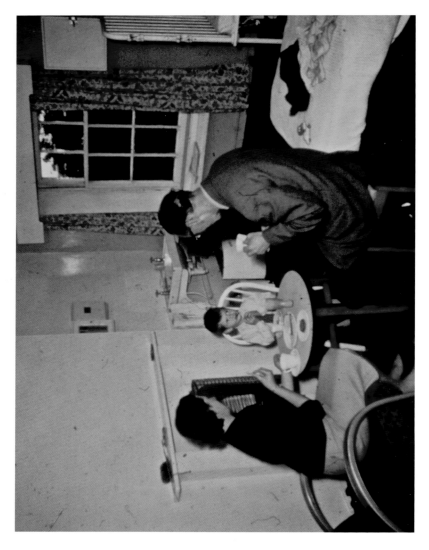

Figure 24: The Babies Hospital at Leazes Terrace 1966
Bed sitting room for mother and child
Audio Visual Centre, Newcastle University

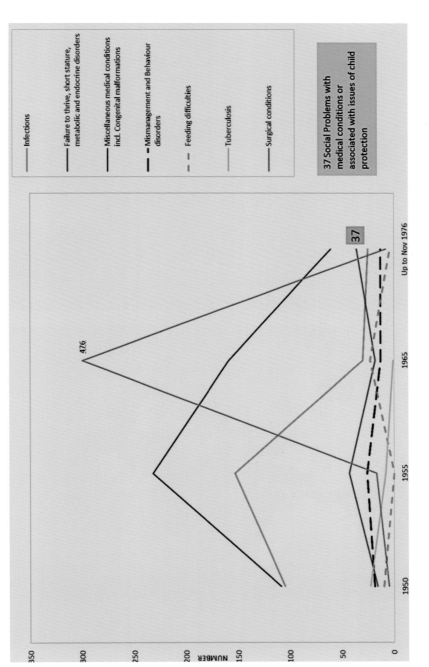

Legend:
- Infections
- Failure to thrive, short stature, metabolic and endocrine disorders
- Miscellaneous medical conditions incl. Congenital malformations
- Mismanagement and Behaviour disorders
- Feeding difficulties
- Tuberculosis
- Surgical conditions

37 Social Problems with medical conditions or associated with issues of child protection

Figure 25: The Babies Hospital at Leazes Terrace. 1950 – November 1976
The changing pattern of diagnoses

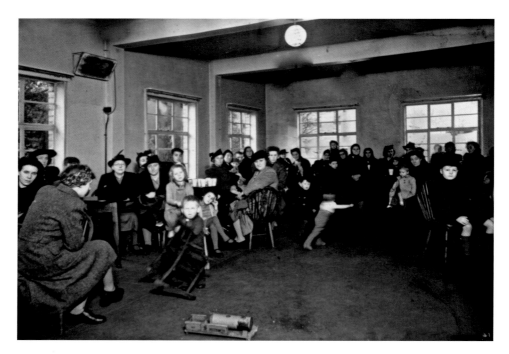

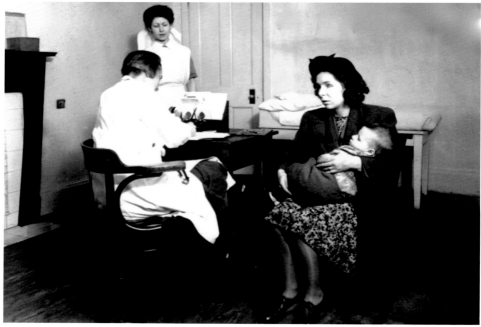

Figures 26a and 26b. The children's clinic. Royal Victoria Infirmary 1946
Photography Department, King's College, Newcastle

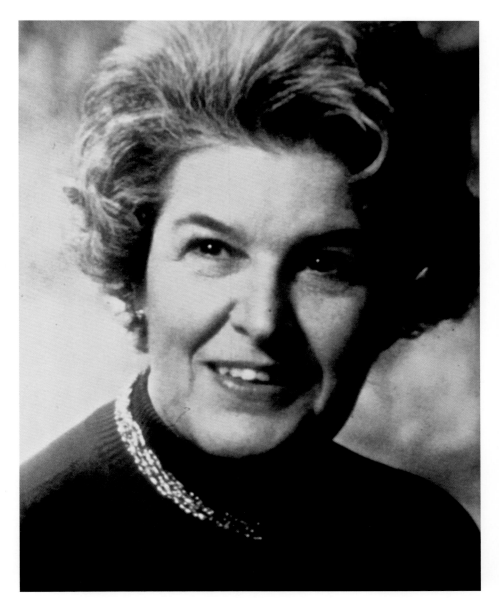

Figure 27: Dr Christine Cooper 1985
Audio Visual Centre, Newcastle University

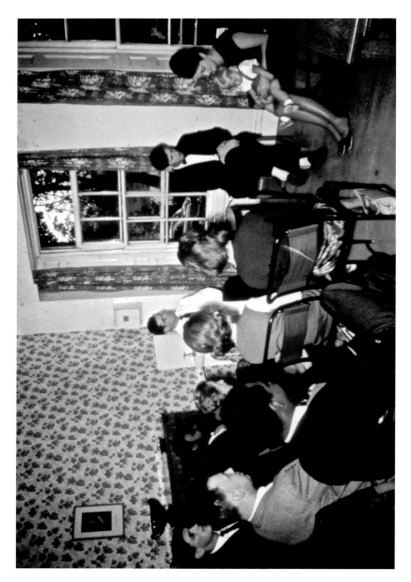

Figure 28: The Babies Hospital, Leazes Terrace 1966
Seminar for students. Dr Michael Parkin is in the white coat
Audio Visual Centre, Newcastle University

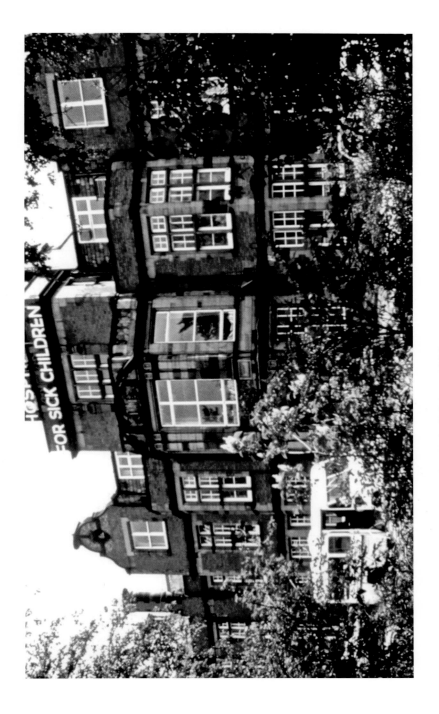

Figure 29: The Fleming Memorial Hospital for Sick Children.1982
Department of photography. Newcastle University

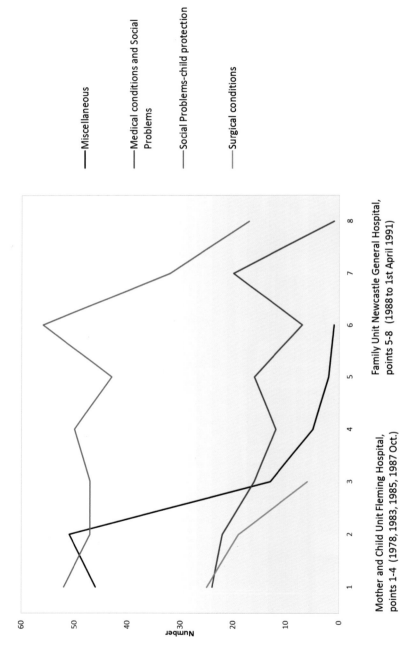

- Miscellaneous
- Medical conditions and Social Problems
- Social Problems-child protection
- Surgical conditions

Mother and Child Unit Fleming Hospital, points 1-4 (1978, 1983, 1985, 1987 Oct.)

Family Unit Newcastle General Hospital, points 5-8 (1988 to 1st April 1991)

Figure 30: The Mother and Child Unit, Fleming Hospital. 1978 – October 1987, and the Family Unit, Newcastle General Hospital. (1988 – 1 April 1991)
The Changing pattern of diagnoses

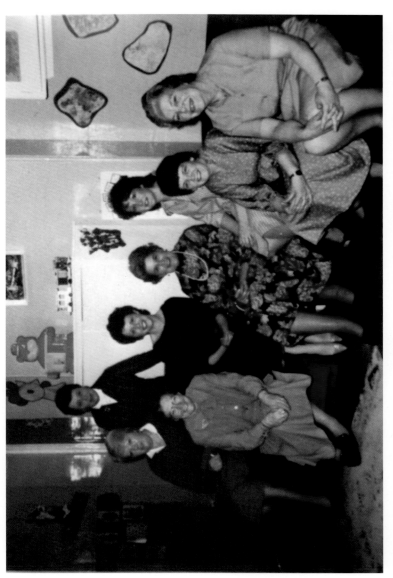

Figure 31: Dr Cooper (centre) at the Mother and Child Unit, Fleming Hospital. 1978. Miss C, Cardose, Nursery Nurse, 3rd from left, Sister E. Greenacre, 2nd from right, Miss A. Matthews, matron, standing on the left Private collection

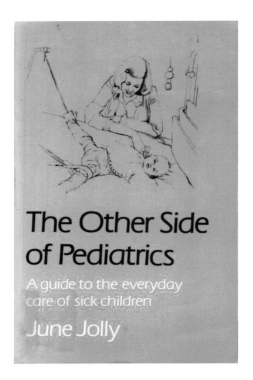

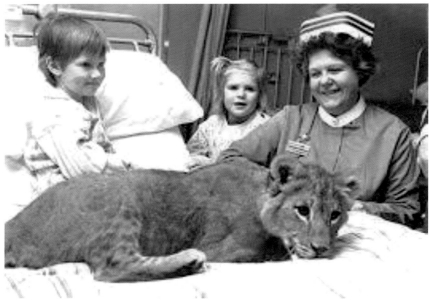

Figure 32. Front cover of a book by June Jolly, 1981 and a photograph in an obituary of her in the Daily Telegraph 12 April 2016.

Family I. A mother and father with their newborn baby

As in the previous case, the father had a history of 'indecency' involving two very young children approximately 3 years ago. This had occurred over a period of time and it appeared that he had not accepted any responsibility for these offences and had consistently denied that they had occurred.

There were also considerable anxieties about the mother's ability to be an effective parent and indeed protect her child in view of limited intellectual abilities, her 'immaturity' and her marked mood changes. The residential assessment was positive in the sense that there was a strong attachment between the parents and the baby and that they were well able to look after her. Mother, however had marked mood swings during which she became restless and angry following minor changes in the daily routine at the Family Unit. During these episodes it was difficult to communicate with her. Her husband appeared to have a calming influence on her.

Notwithstanding the positive features identified in the assessment it was our considered view that there was a considerable risk of harm to the child at the hands of her father and that his wife would not be able to protect her. It was therefore not possible to recommend rehabilitation home. The same multidisciplinary team as in the previous family (Family H) was involved in the assessment. Her child's health, growth and development were normal at that stage.

Comment

These two cases illustrate the considerable anxieties and difficulties that arise when there is a history of sexual abuse of young children by parents or caretakers. The multidisciplinary assessments that were done within a residential setting clarified some of the issues and made a valuable contribution to the recommendations about the future of the children.

Family J. A mother and her two and a half year old toddler

The problems of this family centred around the sexual abuse of this single mother (who was now 23 years old) at the hands of her father over a considerable period of time, starting probably when she was 6 years old; her father was convicted and is currently in prison. She had made a disclosure when her baby was 8 months old. Subsequently, there were considerable problems with marked anxiety, mood swings, depression, irritability and inability to cope with her child. She spent a period of time in a psychiatric hospital but did not have any formal psychiatric illness. At that time, the child was cared for by the maternal grandmother. Subsequently, the increasing demands of her toddler made it very difficult for her to cope and she became anxious that she might harm her and indeed smother her. The child went into foster care and a great deal of individual counselling and help were provided during the time that mother had regular access to her.

By the time the child was two and a half years of age, it was clear that some recommendation had to be made about her long-term future because she was becoming attached to the foster mother. At that time she was in Voluntary Care.

99

A referral was therefore made by the Social Services Department to the Family Unit and over a period of 6 weeks, it was possible to encourage mother to attach to her child more adequately and care for her. She continued to have considerable feelings of anxiety and it was quite clear that she had many unmet needs of her own. Nevertheless, she did begin to look after her daughter quite effectively and she subsequently went home with continuing intense support and help by the community services. Her child's heath, growth and development were normal at that stage.

Family K. A mother and father and their newborn baby
This was the second admission of this family to the Family Unit. Their first child was taken into Care because of physical abuse and has now been adopted. As a result, a residential assessment was undertaken at the Family Unit following the birth of their second child. After that assessment, a recommendation was made for them to return home, but the situation broke down after mother prop fed the baby with a bottle containing very hot fluid, which scalded her mouth. He was therefore taken into foster care. It was also evident that the relationship between the parents was unhappy at the time. A further attempt at rehabilitation was made, but this proved to be unsuccessful.

Following the birth of their third child, the family was once again admitted to the Family Unit. The baby was healthy and normal. They did very well and a multidisciplinary Case Conference recommended that an attempt should be made to support them at home.

This is a most vulnerable family. The mother came from a large family of 8 children with multiple 'psycho-social' problems, unhappy childhood experiences with poor parenting, poor school progress and evidence of considerable immaturity in adolescence. The father already had a 17 year old daughter from a previous marriage which ended in divorce and he has a history of intermittent excessive alcohol intake, poor tolerance to stress and a tendency to follow his own urges. The relationship between the parents, who had known each other for 4 years, had been unstable from time to time, but had improved during recent months. There was little support from the extended family.

It was with a great deal of trepidation that a recommendation was made for this child to go home with his parents. Nevertheless, 3 years later they are doing well and their child is progressing normally.

Comment
This family illustrates the desirability and indeed the necessity of considering afresh the welfare and care of each new child within the family. Some families are able to mature and develop, environmental conditions can improve, relationships with community services can become amicable and some parents can then successfully look after their children with caring support and practical help.

Comment in retrospect (2014)
The history of the plight of successive children at high risk of serious harm, as in this family, Illustrates the dilemmas of the agencies faced with the

duty to protect their safety and welfare. Tolerance and considerable skilled resources have to be deployed over prolonged periods of time. The risks to successive children may vary according to changing circumstances within the family.

NOTE: As in the case of the families assessed at the Mother and Child Unit of the Fleming Memorial Hospital, separate independent reports were written by a child psychologist and psychiatrists who, in this series of cases, participated in the assessments of all these families.

COMMENTARY

During the life of the Babies Hospital (1925-1945), the City of Newcastle upon Tyne had a population close to 300,000. Situated 7 miles along the north bank of the Tyne, it was heavily industrialised. There was considerable unemployment and poverty after the end of the First World War in 1918. Housing was poor with great overcrowding and deficient sanitation, compounded by poor standards of hygiene.[18 Chapter 3] The infant mortality rate was high and in excess of that for England and Wales (Figure 1)

The Annual Reports of the Medical Officer of Health describe the considerable efforts that were made by the City Public Health Department to improve the environmental conditions, the sanitation and the health services for children, pregnant mothers and the rest of the population.

The institutions concerned with health and welfare consisted of Dispensaries as well as Hospitals, Child Welfare Clinics, domiciliary services, including health visitors, Child and Maternal Welfare Medical Officers and general practitioners. There was also a small number of private nursing homes.[18 Chapter 4]

The Royal Victoria Infirmary (RVI), which later became the teaching hospital, and where some children were admitted, was founded in 1777. It was set up by voluntary subscription and remained so until the National Health Service subsumed it in 1948.

The First Childrens Hospital in 1865 in Hanover Square[15] was followed by The Fleming Memorial Hospital For Sick Children in 1887. A new Children's Department was opened at Newcastle General Hospital in 1939. This hospital, which opened in 1870, was the infirmary of the Newcastle Union workhouse and was handed over to the City Council in 1921, under a new Local Government Act. Before 1948, it was a poor law, local authority hospital.[37] In 1943, the Children's Department of the RVI and the Nuffield Clinic at King's College were established. A children's unit developed at Walker Gate Hospital, formerly the Hospital for Infectious Diseases. The Babies Hospital founded in 1925 was unique, compared with all the other hospitals in the City, in that it catered for the youngest sick children under the age of 3 years.

J.C. worked in the era before the availability of antibiotics and sophisticated methods for the investigation of the causes of childhood illness. The requirements were high standards of basic nursing care, attention to hygiene and adequate nutrition including an emphasis on natural breastfeeding, adequate rest and fresh air. Massage was also available for some children with mental as well as physical disabilities.

The origins of Sir James Spence's legacy may be traced to his appointment in Newcastle in 1923 as Honorary Medical Officer to a day nursery in a poor, socially deprived area of the city. Before his arrival, a high prevalence of ill health, poor nutrition, inadequate home care and lack of adequate services for the young children of that community had already been documented. Adverse family and social factors affecting their health and welfare had also been identified.

A decision had therefore been made to allocate a section of the nursery to cater mainly for the nutritional problems of babies and infants on a residential basis. These problems were at the root of much of the ill health in this age group and hospital services in Newcastle and the northern districts were deficient in their ability and capacity to cater for them. Accommodation, nursing skills and medical and surgical expertise were limited for the provision of the most effective care for this age group. J.C. led the development of a full-scale Babies Hospital after the closure of the West End Day Nursery in 1924.

It was an era when very sick babies were not given any priority for treatment in some quarters, because it seemed that so little could be done for them. Across the United Kingdom, children under the age of 2 years were seldom admitted to some hospitals during the early years of the 20th century. There were also concerns about cross-infection and the deleterious effects of separation from their mothers. Visiting by parents was positively discouraged because it was the belief that it upset the children. J.C. wrote eloquently about the fallacy of excluding the youngest from hospital treatment in order to prevent the survival of infants in poor health so as to ensure a healthy population; he pointed out that inclusive health services for all age groups are associated with a healthier population in adulthood. In some instances, as in the case of infants with tuberculosis, there was virtually no other suitable accommodation anywhere else in Newcastle and the northern districts. For the life-threatening conditions during that era of pyloric stenosis, hare lip and cleft palate, an expert service was not readily available elsewhere for the surgery and the special requirements of pre- and post-operative care.

Unlike the earlier hospitals for children, which originated in Britain during the second half of the 19th century, the Babies Hospital was not established specifically to cater for the 'deserving' poor. During the Victorian period, families on relief associated with the Poor Law were:

"Denied attendance at the new paediatric hospitals on the principle that they were already recipients of public aid," and "to ensure that only the deserving poor were served, a subscriber's letter of recommendation was usually required before a child could be admitted either as an outpatient or as an inpatient."[36]

At the Babies Hospital, payment was sought only for the inpatient treatment of a relatively small number of private patients. After 1927, this amounted to about 6% of the total annual income and involved only about 5% of admissions during the years before the Second World War. Additional unspecified fees were also paid to the doctors.

The hospital was located in a poor area of Newcastle and its origin in a day nursery was a response to specific needs arising from the social conditions during and after the First World War. Initially, the plight of the children of munitions workers attracted attention. Later, it included the ill health identified as a direct result of the medical examination of children attending the nursery and the increasing knowledge of the needs of their mothers and families.

From the outset, the hospital had the active support of the Newcastle City Public Health Department, which had taken significant steps to alleviate the ill health and high infant mortality and lower birth rate of the late 19th and early 20th centuries. It did not rely on the exclusive patronage of wealthy individuals, some of whom in the past had been intent on promoting their social standing whilst benefitting the community. There were none of the Victorian oppositions based on moral objections of undermining family responsibilities, objections from physicians seeking protection of their financial interests and concerns that children would not thrive without their parents.

Referrals to the Babies Hospital for inpatient treatment were made by doctors from child welfare clinics and general practice. Decisions to admit for inpatient treatment were made by the honorary medical staff mainly in outpatients clinics held at the hospital. The criteria were based strictly on clinical priorities. The Victorian practice of admission on the recommendation of subscribers was not in place. The hospital relied in part on funding from the Ministry of Health during the early years and local authorities as well as public donations throughout its life. Very few families paid for the service for their children.

The particulars of James Spence's involvement in the hospital's care of sick children provide a new insight into his legacy. It was a time when paediatrics and child health became a well-established branch of medicine. He was a pioneer in the development of the speciality in Newcastle and wider afield over a period of over 20 years (1924-1945) at the Babies Hospital. His work also led to a greater understanding by the medical profession and the public of the physical, emotional and social needs of children and their families.

Through the prism of a complete set of Annual Reports from the Babies Hospital in which he compiled the medical components, he documented the diseases and disorders of the inpatients treated at the hospital and the immediate outcome. He shed light on the nature and treatment of their disorders and the latest research about causes, prevention and best available care. As a result of his perceptive commentaries, a vivid narrative emerges like a voice from the past, about the ideas and priorities that led to further improvements in the understanding of childhood disease, the treatment of the youngest children in Newcastle and the northern districts and eventually to the groundbreaking researches into the family and social factors that determine the survival, health and welfare of children and their families.

His early initiative to invite mothers to come into residence with their sick children in a homely and welcoming environment, in order to care for them under the guidance of the nursing staff, was made primarily on pragmatic grounds. It remains a landmark element of his legacy. It led to a great improvement in care and was life-saving in some cases; the outcome in surgical cases was particularly positive. When mothers were unable to come into residence because of family or other pressing commitments, they were invited to come in daily to take part in their children's care. They were encouraged to breastfeed if at all

104

possible and learn about their care. For many years, the name of the hospital was 'The Babies Hospital and Mothercraft Centre'.

J.C. indicated that sentiment did not play a part in the provisions for mothers. He and the nursing staff nevertheless quickly came to appreciate the great personal and clinical benefits to the children, the mothers and the entire service. It was in sharp contrast during that era to the stark environment of paediatric wards in the main hospitals, with parents' access to their children severely restricted and the lack of participation of the mothers in their care. As late as 1946, in the Charles West Lecture on the care of children in hospital, J.C. described a memorable, most disturbing portrayal of the state of children's wards in many hospitals in the country and the deprivations and distress of the children (Appendix 4)[27]. A new, more humane ethos of hospital care of children was established. As Professor Court pointed out, J.C. had an "intuitive understanding of people"[10], no doubt reinforced by his numerous contacts in his outpatient clinics and private practice. He took practical steps to apply these insights to the care of children in hospital.

Malnutrition and severe wasting were the dominant clinical states encountered during the early years of the hospital. They were associated with infections, as yet undiagnosed medical conditions, inappropriate feeding, late diagnosis of pyloric stenosis and inadequate early home-care of hare lip and cleft palate. The special nursing skills that were developed to care for these children were the foundation for the reputation of the hospital as a model for the care of sick babies and infants. The origins of J.C.'s legacy in relation to the promotion of breast feeding and adequate nutrition may be traced to these early clinical experiences at the West End Nursery and Babies Hospital and Mothercraft Centre.

As marasmus gave way to specific diagnoses of organic diseases, there evolved a distinctive pattern of diseases and disorders treated at the hospital. Priority was given to severe infections alongside the hazardous surgical conditions of pyloric stenosis, hare lip and cleft palate. Some degree of malnutrition, often severe, was usually a contributory factor to the clinical problems.

The skills of the physicians were an essential element of pre- and post-operative care. J.C. left a legacy of close collaboration and 'conference' with the surgeons, which resulted in excellent outcomes for that era. Even Lady Ridley, who was still chair of the Management Committee, took sole charge of the operating theatre at Blagdon Hall during the war years and assisted at most operations, when many trained nurses were called up at the outbreak of hostilities.[3] She herself had no training in nursing.

The successful operative treatment of hare lip and cleft palate, allied to the outpatient care with speech therapy, were pioneering activities that attained widespread national and international attention. J.C. also ensured that there were excellent amicable relationships between the medical, surgical and nursing staff, the matron and the members of the Management Committee of the hospital. This is an early indication of the 'collegiate' spirit of friendship that he fostered thereafter with everyone in the Children's Department in Newcastle. It led eventually to his famous statement on welcoming Dr Donald Court to a research post in 1946:

"The first aim of my department is comradeship, not achievement."[4]

He also promoted close collaboration with public bodies, which ensured their continuing support, including the finances, throughout the life of the hospital.

As Professor Court pointed out in 1975 in an assessment of J.C.'s legacy, it is a result of the epidemiological studies that he initiated in Newcastle, that he made the connections between infection, nutrition and social environment.[10] The insights that he gained from his clinical experiences at the Babies Hospital played an important part in the genesis of these studies[18, 39, 40,41-46] and the orientation of paediatrics towards the environmental and social imperatives that contribute to the health and welfare of children and their families.

A special feature of the hospital was a strong presence of women on the Management Committee. A few were titled, with Lady Ridley in the chair for most of the life of the hospital, but most came from the middle classes. This was in contrast to other children's hospitals in Britain where men were almost exclusively in charge. J.C. himself recommended several women to join the committee of the hospital.[8]

During the inter-war years, the hospital acquired a national and international reputation for the innovative care and successful medical and surgical treatment of sick babies and infants. J.C. recommended that distinctive inpatient arrangements, separate to those for older children and adults, have to be made to meet the needs of sick babies and infants and their resident mothers.

The total number admitted every year to the Babies Hospital was relatively small, and only a modest proportion of the sick children of that age group in Newcastle and the northern districts who required inpatient treatment could be accommodated. Nevertheless, all the available information about the work of the Babies Hospital from that era allows for an informative narrative of the legacy of J.C. to the health care and welfare of children and the advances in knowledge and provision of hospital care for them.

J.C. belonged to an era when the consultant physician for children was a generalist who assumed responsibility for all age groups and the treatment of all their diseases. He wrote about the need for physicians to be expert in the field of children's diseases. He believed in the value of specialists but did not accept the autonomy of sub-specialisation in community medicine. He was unwilling to recognise a differentiation between this speciality and clinical and laboratory medicine. He encouraged the doctors that he appointed to take a special interest and acquire expertise in some of the conditions that were encountered. For example, Dr Gerald Neligan (First Assistant) became an expert on osteitis,[8] Dr H. Jackson (Research Associate in the 1000 Families Study) an authority on childhood accidents and Dr F.J.W. Miller a leading expert on childhood tuberculosis. There was however no attempt to develop comprehensive sub-specialisation during his lifetime.

He expected hospital doctors to enter the community from time to time as "field workers" to study the prevalent diseases.[97] This occurred in the pioneering 1000 Families Study in Newcastle. It was not until two decades after the closure of the first Babies Hospital in 1945 that sub-specialisation in paediatrics was widely accepted in Newcastle.[98] He did however leave a legacy of active involvement of paediatricians in the problems relating to the health and welfare of children and their families in the communities of Newcastle and the northern region. Two decades after his death this led to active participation in child protection and the involvement of consultant paediatricians in the clinical services and multidisciplinary activities in the community, with specialisation in other areas such as chronic disability and mental health.

In addition to his views about the organisation within the hospital, he urged paediatricians to "make themselves expert in the physical examination of institutions" in order to provide the most effective services for children.[27] In the early 1930s, he was already planning for a modern children's hospital to accommodate all the paediatric wards and outpatient clinics of the city. The provisions would include accommodation for all mothers, who were able to participate in the care of their children. These proposals were not realised until after 2009 when a purpose-built children's hospital, the Great North Children's Hospital, was opened at the RVI. Every parent can now stay with their child and families can also be accommodated in a separate house on the site of the hospital. This is a significant improvement on the residential capacity at the original Babies Hospital, in which about a third of the children were admitted with their mothers by 1944. However, the ideal promoted by J.C. of every mother sharing a comfortable room with her baby and infant with sufficient space, privacy and amenities has not yet been realised in some children's hospitals nationwide. The current arrangements in many paediatric wards of parents sleeping on pull-down beds or an unused patient's bed, sometimes for prolonged periods, are unsatisfactory. There is considerable discomfort and distress to parents who may be "exhausted, and reduced to tears by sleep deprivation and the lack of privacy." Although there are excellent facilities for parents in many hospitals including in Newcastle, financial considerations in the National Health Service are now the main constraint on the provision of more appropriate facilities.[99]

Over the years, J.C. insisted on the importance of research and by 1938 had raised sufficient funds to set up a Clinical Research Department at the Babies Hospital, supported by the Medical Research Council. He made important contributions to knowledge about the nature and treatment of organic disease in childhood and the family, social and environmental conditions, which determine the health and welfare of children and their families. These are detailed in a bibliography of all his writings in the 'The Purpose and Practice of Medicine'.[4] In one specific instance - Pink Disease - he, like everyone else in paediatrics, completely failed to find the cause despite taking a special interest in the condition and conducting some research. His forte was also the logical application of all the knowledge that was available, the provision of the most appropriate and humane hospital arrangements for the treatment of sick children and the dissemination of the fruits of his knowledge and experience to the medical profession and the public. He expected his staff to develop specific expertise in the diseases that came to the fore during that era.

The extensive teaching at the Babies Hospital for medical students and postgraduates was the forerunner of the courses and attachments to the paediatric wards of the main hospitals following the development of a new curriculum for paediatrics at the medical school in Newcastle. The training of probationers and nurses was also an important contribution to the care of babies and infants in the community in the City and the northern region.

J.C. was by all accounts a memorable teacher, who left a legacy of unforgettable examples of his ingenuity. Professor Court wrote that he was "always a teacher" and capable of:

"Painting a vivid portrait of child and disease in the 20 minutes he allowed himself for a clinical lecture, sensitively releasing the hidden fears of a mother in outpatient consultation, and in lively conversation over tea in the department with staff and visitors."[10]

Dr Kurt Schapira, who was a medical student in Newcastle in 1946 and later a prominent consultant psychiatrist in the city, and a notable raconteur, recalls several instances of J.C.'s teaching methods.[100]

On a ward round at the Royal Victoria Infirmary, a group of students stood at the bedside of a young boy. J.C. asked them to describe the lesion on his forearm; the size, shape, surface, colour, depth on palpation, the presence of discomfort or pain, the appearance of the arm and general appearance of the child. He then asked whether there was anything else that might be investigated. One student, an older man who had recently served in the armed services during the war, suggested that perhaps they should elicit whether the lesion had a smell. Without batting an eyelid, J.C. asked him to kneel down at the bedside and perform the test. He asked him to describe his findings. The reply was that there was no smell. Whereupon J.C. commented in words to the effect: "There you are gentlemen, this man who had never seen such a lesion before and had no knowledge of its significance, has made a new discovery and now knows more about a tuberculin reaction than I ever did after many years of clinical practice."

On another occasion, a group of students gathered at the cot-side of a child sitting there in obvious distress, making a loud noise with his laboured breathing. J.C. had not seen the child before and had not been given any account of the history at that stage. He asked them to describe what they saw and heard and eventually elicited the observation of a 'stridor'. He then asked them what should be done about it – silence – so, as he stood at the side of the cot, he leaned over and observed the child closely for a few seconds and then gave him a mighty pat on the back. The child coughed and up came a piece of apple with immediate relief of symptoms.

Dr John Walton (later Lord Walton of Detchant), who had been his house physician at the RVI following an undergraduate career in Newcastle during the Second World War, also commented on J.C.'s "virtuosity and inspiration"[101a] and his "universally exciting ward rounds, despite some of his unusual ideas", when many visitors from elsewhere in the UK and overseas joined his teaching sessions. He witnessed the incident of the expulsion of the foreign body from the toddler's chest, but records it to have been a pea rather than a piece of apple![101b]

Colleagues who had worked closely with him during the 1930s and 1940s have written "like all good teachers he exaggerated"[8] and "the outpatient sessions at West Parade were visited by many discerning students."[7b]

Although J.C. was very popular with students and colleagues, there were times when he irritated some of them by his unusual and challenging approach. Dr Fred Miller who was one of the honorary assistant physicians at the Babies Hospital following his appointment in 1938 as senior child welfare medical officer in Newcastle and who had the greatest respect for him, wrote in his memoir:

"Although I was strongly attracted by Spence's personality, the students as a group were sharply divided into those who admired him and others who did not and called him James "Clever" Spence."[7b]

Dr Dick Ellis who was his registrar, then his first assistant for many years and later one of the consultant paediatricians in Newcastle, recalled occasions when colleagues became frustrated during ward rounds at the RVI when J.C. was inclined to 'pontificate' without giving an opinion or any practical help.[8]

During the penultimate year of the Babies Hospital in 1944, J.C. recorded in the Annual Report the principal lessons that he had learnt about clinical practice and hospital organisation. The admission of mothers to care for their sick children was welcomed and eventually accepted universally. On the other hand, his contention that physicians should be responsible for the day-to-day care of the children and the organisation in a combined medical and surgical ward, was not accepted by the paediatric surgeons who were later appointed to the Children's Department in Newcastle.[102]

The Babies Hospital provided him with important elements of clinical, administrative, educational and research experience that contributed to his appointment in Newcastle in 1942 as the first fulltime Professor of Child Health in England. He then took every opportunity to promote training, research into the prevention, causes and treatment of childhood diseases and the provision of services appropriate to the special requirements of children of all ages. As a result, his counsel was sought widely in Newcastle, the northern region and at a national and international level.

On the advent of the National Health Service, his legacy was maintained in a new Babies Hospital for a further 28 years (1948 -1976) by paediatricians that he himself had appointed, including Dr Gerald Neligan, Dr Christine Cooper and his successor, Professor Donald Court. Extensive changes took place during those years in the nature of the conditions investigated and treated at the hospital. This was the result of the decline in infectious diseases requiring hospital treatment, the identification and treatment of an increasing range of organic diseases and surgical conditions that could be treated. There was also the development of sub-specialities such as paediatric cardiology and the introduction into the hospital of children with developmental, behavioural and management problems. The ambience, with accommodation for mothers and a ready access to fathers and other family members, was maintained.

During the final year of the hospital in 1976, there is a record of yet a further group of children who came to the attention of paediatricians. They had been abused or badly cared for by their parents or caretakers and came in with their mothers for an assessment of their condition and the causes of any problems within their family and environment. This took place in order to make recommendations about their future care and the possibility of supporting and helping their families in the community.

Child protection became a new priority for paediatrics during the late 1960s and early 1970s and after the closure of the Babies Hospital at Leazes Terrace, further residential hospital facilities were set aside in Newcastle over the next 20 years (1977-1997) to cater for help and a thorough assessment of vulnerable families with child protection issues. The paediatric wards in the main hospitals were just not suited to this purpose and residential facilities were provided in the Mother and Child Unit of the Fleming Memorial Hospital for Sick Children (1977-1986) and the Family Unit at Newcastle General Hospital (1988-1997). J.C.'s legacy persisted for 43 years after his death.

J.C. and his colleagues had identified 'problem families' in Newcastle about 15 years earlier in the Thousand Families Study of 1947. The presence in the community of children who had been abused and neglected was recognised, as were some of the 'psycho-social' factors that afflicted these families.[18] Knowledge of the causes and how to deal with the problems, however were limited and multidisciplinary systems for child protection had not yet evolved between social services and paediatrics, child psychology and psychiatry, community health and education services,

Amongst the paediatricians of Newcastle, it was Dr Christine Cooper who had been J.C.'s senior registrar and was greatly influenced by his empathy and understanding of the needs of children and families in the community, who initiated the service for the assessment, support and protection of these vulnerable children and their families. Her background, training and contributions to child protection are described in some detail because she made such vital contributions to the identification, prevention and management of these disturbing problems. Her dedication and dogged determination were legendary. She was amongst the first paediatricians in the country to pay attention to these new priorities.

Dr Cooper also wrote persuasively about "good-enough parenting",[62] "babies at risk"[74] and "seeing the baby after the birth by mothers, who were renouncing them for adoption."[103]

After 1968, she was greatly influenced by the tragic events in Newcastle upon Tyne that year surrounding the manslaughter of two boys aged 3 and 4 years by Mary Bell (age 11 years), who strangled the boys in Scotswood, an inner-city suburb of the west end of the city.[104, 105, 106] Dr Cooper had a brief involvement earlier in the child's life. She was the first child of her 17 year old mother, who was a prostitute often away in Glasgow. The identity of her father was not known. The first reaction of her mother immediately after her birth in the maternity hospital was to "take the thing away from me."[105] Her mother later married a habitual criminal who had also committed an armed robbery. Her extended family believed that the mother had tried to kill her on several occasions and made it look like accidents. Mary maintained that she had been sexually abused from the age of 4 years by men forced on her by her mother. She was an intelligent girl who had a lonely, troubled childhood devoid of affection.

Dr Cooper had been involved in the child's case as indicated by the following record registered at Newcastle General Hospital seven years before Mary's conviction:

"Mary Flora Bell, 28, Elswick Road, Newcastle upon Tyne 6/3/61 to 9/3/61: under care of consultant Dr Cooper."[106]

She was familiar with psycho-analytic theories and also accepted the principles defined by Bowlby that 'real events' rather than the 'fantasy' of 'internal life' of infants, as suggested by these theories, were the driving elements in later emotional and personality development and that children's experiences of interpersonal relationships were crucial to their psychological development.[107] These principles informed her work and that of her successors at the hospital units that continued to provide assessments as part of the multi-disciplinary services for 'vulnerable' children and families for three decades after these events. There was also a recognition that emotional abuse occurred in varying degrees in all other forms of abuse and was the predominant affliction in some children.[108]

The other case which had a considerable impact on her was that of Maria Colwell who was killed in 1973 by her stepfather. She was placed in foster care early in her life, when she was a "happy normal little girl." On returning to live with her mother, a new partner with several children of his own rejected her. Neighbours and teachers raised concerns, which were ignored. In the end, she died with severe internal and brain injuries, a "living skeleton."[109]

The plight of this child led to fundamental changes in the law relating to child care. From the outset, Dr Cooper was actively involved in the national discussions amongst paediatricians which followed the tragedy. Plans were made for the study, prevention, appropriate assessment and care of suspected abuse and neglect.[59] The NSPCC and DHSS were also involved at an early stage. One of the consequences was the greater involvement of paediatricians in the assessment and support of vulnerable children and their families. Attitudes towards the protection of children in Britain had been evolving for 100 years since the 1870s.[110] A series of Children Acts enshrined new policies and practices between 1908 and 1989, from greater child orientation in 1908 to the establishment of local authorities in 1948 with a new emphasis on restoration of the care of children to their parents in preference to residential homes and better arrangements for adoption. J.C. was a member of the Curtis Committee in 1946[111] that made the recommendations in the 1948 Act.

The 1975 Children Act was largely a response to the Maria Colwell tragedy. Substitute care became the guiding principle when care within the 'natural', biological family was inadequate. By 1989, the balance in the Act of that year shifted still further by replacing the concept of the 'rights and duties' of parents with 'parental responsibilities' as the primary focus for child protection. Support for children and families and a partnership between parents and local health, social and educational services were to be promoted, as well as more thorough multidisciplinary assessments of families. An important consequence of the Act was a diminishing role of the hospital based paediatric service that had evolved in Newcastle to participate in the assessment and support of vulnerable children and their families. Eventually, it contributed to the demise of the service as it moved into the community.

During the early life of the Babies Hospital under J.C., priority was given to babies with pyloric stenosis and hare lip and cleft palate, who probably would not have survived without hospital treatment. Five decades later, priority was also given to babies who were at serious risk of harm and even death, not because of any organic disorder, but because of abuse and neglect at the hands of their parents and caretakers. The arrangements initiated by J.C. for the residence of mothers to participate in the care of their children in a separate and appropriate hospital environment were still welcomed to cater for these newly identified problems

It is of historical interest that J.C. did not accept the insights of Psychology and Psychiatry about the mental health of children. This is recorded in 1975 by Professor Court in his evaluation of J.C.'s legacy.[10] It may have contributed to a delay in the establishment of a Psychology and Psychiatry Department for children and young people in Newcastle until the 1960s. There was also a prolonged delay during J.C.'s lifetime in allowing mothers to come into residence or visit them without restrictions, when their children (mainly over the age of 3 years) were admitted to the paediatric wards of the main hospitals in Newcastle. The adverse emotional effects would have been particularly damaging in the very young under the age of 3 years, who were suddenly, uncomprehendingly left in the care of strangers with the additional stresses of a very restricted routine of visiting by mothers and family members. Older children would also have been affected.

This was the norm in the paediatric wards nationwide during the first half of the 20th century. J.C.'s Babies Hospital was a notable exception, where mothers were resident and made welcome as early as 1924. In 1951, an inquiry by the Ministry of Health revealed that out of the 1300 hospitals in Britain that admitted children, only 300 allowed daily visiting, usually limited to 30 minutes. 150 prohibited visiting altogether.[112]

There is thus a puzzling discrepancy between the welcoming arrangements for mothers at the Babies Hospital and the severe restrictions of visiting and a lack of residential facilities for them in the paediatric wards of the main hospitals in Newcastle, as at the RVI where J.C had consultant responsibilities. Very young children under the age of 5 years were also inpatients in these wards, in which these deficiencies persisted for many years.

Professor Court wrote in 1975:

"As the gifted amateur suspects the professional, so his intuitive understanding of people made him unwilling to recognise the extent and

112

complexity of mental ill health in children and resistant to the development of child psychiatry as an independent discipline." [10]

Fourteen years later in 1989, a new insight came to light as a result of a description of several encounters between J.C. and Dr James Robertson, a psychologist and trained psychoanalyst from the Tavistock Clinic in London. The circumstances and consequences are not generally known. The authors of the present study were not aware of them during their long association with the Department of Child Health in Newcastle. Disturbing examples of potentially damaging inpatient care of young children had been identified by Dr Robertson in hospitals in Britain. These encounters are now described in detail in order to attempt to clarify the issues as they reflect on elements of J.C.'s legacy. The account is taken directly from that published by Dr Robertson and his wife Joyce, 38 years after these meetings had taken place. [113]

In 1951, at the suggestion of Dr Alan Moncrieff from Great Ormond Street Hospital, Dr Robertson was invited by the British Paediatric Association (BPA) to present the results of three years of detailed day by day observations of the behaviour of very young children admitted to hospital paediatric wards without their mothers and very limited contact with them during their inpatient treatment. This was part of a systematic inquiry into the effects on personality development of separation from the mother in early childhood. The presentation took place at the Annual Meeting of the BPA at Windermere in the presence of most of the prominent paediatricians of the day.

Dr Robertson described the consistent observations of three most distressing conditions that rapidly took hold of the children on the wards. He decided to name these as a sequence of 'Protest, Despair and Detachment'. In some of the children that he observed in their homes after discharge from hospital, he noted adverse behaviour, including:

"Clinging to the mother, temper tantrums, disturbed sleep, bedwetting, regression and aggression particularly against the mother as if blaming her."

He went on to describe the immediate response of the paediatricians who heard his account, concentrating specifically on J.C.'s reaction, who was at that time one of the leading paediatricians in the country. He had been knighted the year before for his services for children and was president of the BPA that year.

J.C. was the first delegate to respond and Dr Robertson records:

"To my extreme dismay, Spence stood up in the large gathering and sweepingly attacked me in a fluent and biting vein of irony. This tall distinguished-looking man, whom I respected, referred dismissingly to what I had said about 'emotional upset' in young patients in hospital. 'What is wrong with emotional upset? This year we are celebrating the centenary of the year of the birth of Wordsworth, the great Lakeland Poet. He suffered from emotional upset, yet look at the poems he produced."

113

Dr Robertson expected J.C. "to be an ally." He goes on to record that other "paediatricians were considerate of me, but no one appeared lit up by my concerns."

After a short while, still upset and puzzled by J.C.'s unexpected response at the BPA, he called on him unexpectedly in Newcastle, where he met with a friendly welcome. He goes on to record their discussions:

"It became clear that I had been a whipping-boy for his antipathy towards psychiatrists. He spoke scathingly about psychiatry, which in his view fragmented people's individuality so that the essential person was lost sight of. He talked about his belief that every paediatrician should not only have a concern for the entire family but should express this by doing home visits and carrying the responsibility unaided. Spence would not employ a psychiatrist or social worker; his paediatric registrars were taught to be respectful and courteous to child patients and their parents and to hold family units together. He thought me sincere but misguided in being associated with a psychiatric clinic."

He was then taken on a tour of the Babies Hospital and the paediatric wards of one of the main hospitals nearby, where J.C. also had consultant responsibilities. At the Babies Hospital, he was most impressed by the welcome accorded to mothers and their intimate involvement in the care of their children, with frequent visiting when they were unable to be resident. In complete contrast, on the paediatric wards of the main hospital where young children were also treated for urgent illnesses and accidents, there were no residential facilities and visiting was restricted to twice a week only (a total of two hours) and he relates that "I immediately detected there the phenomena of Protest and Despair that I had seen elsewhere."

He asked J.C. to reconcile these striking differences and recorded:

"He patted my knee as if to comfort me in my unnecessary concern," and said, "Robertson, I know how much these children need. Twice a week is enough."

He also records his own reaction:

"It struck me forcibly that kindness, however genuine, was no substitute for understanding the emotional needs of infants and young children."

Also:

"An enormous meshing of defences against acknowledging the distress and psychological deterioration in young patients."

He had already observed in other hospitals that the provisions for inpatient treatment included the imperatives of an orderly, quiet, tidy ward environment in which the nurses could take care of the children 'efficiently'. However, these circumstances did not allow them to spend time comforting and mothering them as would be done naturally by their parents or playing with them. The children who were well enough to move about or walk were usually let out of their cots for a while to a play room, but the others were often left in their cots for the entire day. In addition there was still a widespread belief that children would be further upset by frequent contact with their non-resident parents who might also bring and spread infections into the wards. The fact that the staff was discouraged to provide one to one care and even cuddle the children was also common in that era, compounded, as suggested by Dr Robertson, by a general suppression of the feelings of 'pain' by the doctors and nurses witnessing daily the inevitable distress of the children under their care. It was also the general belief that a 'quiet' child was a 'happy' child.

It was a direct result of the resistance of J.C. and the health professions to acknowledge the deprivations of young children in hospital and the failure to improve their conditions, that Dr James Robertson with his wife Joyce, who had participated in his researches over many years, embarked on filming the behaviour of unaccompanied children in hospitals, nurseries and foster care.[113] These were a potent source of the improvements that eventually took place in the care of children in hospital.

Dr Robertson recorded two further encounters with J.C. around 1952-1953. He writes:

"I returned to Newcastle and a large staff meeting presided over by Professor Spence. I thought that since my film ('A Two-year-old Goes to Hospital') was an objective and non-critical record the professor would give it his blessing. But my wishful expectations of appreciative acceptance were dashed. After the showing he was as caustically negative as before and his lieutenants followed his lead."

"When a few months later we flew together to a seminar in Paris, he told me he preferred the simple if misguided honesty of my orientation to the 'more dangerous attitudes' of Dr Bowlby. And it seemed that despite the invulnerability of his rejection of my views there was a touch of conscience."

It is of interest that a pivotal report by Dr John Bowlby, entitled "Maternal Care and Mental Health"[114] published during the same year as J.C.'s first encounter with Dr Robertson, referred approvingly to J.C.'s seminal lectures in 1946 on "The Purpose of the Family"[52] (The Convocation Lecture to the National Children's Home) and "The Care of Children In Hospital"[27] (The Charles West Lecture), in which he demonstrated a thorough knowledge of the development and needs of children.

Dr Bowlby was a senior colleague of Dr Robertson and the Director of the Child Guidance Department at the Tavistock Clinic. This most influential report was commissioned by the World Health Organisation (WHO) in response to a decision by the Social Commission of the United Nation in 1948 to study the needs of homeless children in their own country. WHO offered to study the mental aspects of the problem.

The children included those in day nurseries, institutions and hospitals (especially those providing long-term care).

Dr Bowlby writing about the conditions that are essential for the prevention of deprivation referred to J.C.'s:

"Inspiring lecture, carrying a title ('The Purpose of the Family') which has been borrowed to name this chapter, one of the principal purposes of the family is the preservation of the art of parenthood."

Furthermore, on reviewing the literature and meeting with many concerned with child care and child guidance, he observed that the understanding that mental health was dependent on the quality of life in the earliest years of the child's life came:

"First from the psycho-analytic treatment of adults and then from that of children...greatly amplified by psychologists and psychiatrists in child guidance clinics and child care."

Paediatricians had not played a part in this process, but he pointed out in relation to the separation of sick children from their families on admission to hospital:

"Leading paediatricians in many countries – among them Spence and Moncrieff in Britain – are alive to the problem, but there remains a great lag in reform."

Highlighting J.C.'s contributions, Bowlby refers to the Charles West Lecture of 1946 in which J.C. gives a comprehensive account of the requirements of a children's hospital to meet the needs of treatment and the appropriate care of the children and their families. He commended the arrangements and practices at the Babies Hospital initiated and developed by J.C. as of fundamental importance to the genesis of his vision of a modern service.

"In those cases where children must come into hospital much can be done to minimise the emotional shock. In the case of children under three, Spence has long advocated whenever possible the admission of the mother with the baby."

We recognise now that this applied almost entirely only to the relatively small number of children admitted to the Babies Hospital. Furthermore, his original reason in 1925 for encouraging mothers to come into residence with their sick children was strictly pragmatic, in order to complement the practical care of the nurses, which could be life-saving particularly in surgical cases. He made it clear at that stage that 'sentiment' did not come into consideration. As is indicated below, it was not until later that he explicitly demonstrated his understanding of the emotional needs of children and that practical measures had to be taken to cater for their needs as inpatients according to their age and

116

stage of development. There was some provision for resident mothers on the paediatric wards of NGH, but none at the RVI and FMH in 1951.

Bowlby was no doubt influenced in this apparent mistaken view of the arrangements for the majority of children admitted to the paediatric wards of the main hospitals in Newcastle, in which mothers were not in residence and visiting was severely restricted, by his appreciation of J.C.'s account of his experiences as a member of the Curtis Committee during 1944-1946, when he was able to observe at first hand the plight of children in many institutions and hospitals in Britain. He was impressed by J.C.'s:

"Vivid picture of deprivation in children's wards, fully as bad as those to be found in the worst of the large institutions now universally condemned. He refers especially to the isolation, aimlessness, and uncertainty of children in long-stay hospitals."

There is a memorable account by J.C. in the Charles West Lecture of 1946 of the awful conditions that he had encountered in a 'typical' paediatric ward during those years; this includes the lack of accommodation for mothers. A transcript is recorded in Appendix 4.

He attributed responsibility for this state of affairs to:

"Usually in a failure to define personal responsibility, or in the imposition of personal responsibility by a remote governing or administrative body on a staff, who are unwilling to confess or complain about their difficulties."

J.C. concludes by making detailed suggestions for improvements. These consist of the staffing requirements, the equipment, the physical arrangements and the administration of the ward. He advocates the residence of mothers to participate in the nursing care of their children in a special suite of rooms close to the wards, in order to participate in the care of their children under the guidance of the nursing staff. However, as in the case in his commentaries in the Annual Reports from the Babies Hospital, he does not refer explicitly to the emotional needs of the children and has no comments on arrangements for visiting when the parents are not in residence. His detailed description of a typical children's ward during that era indicates, however, that he had an acute awareness of the emotional distress of the unaccompanied children and he expresses implicitly his own distress in what he had observed in those wards. In relation to children in 'special' (fever) hospitals, he comments:

"If at times we tend to neglect the comfort and emotional welfare of the children in these institutions by leaving that responsibility to others, we are quickly brought back to reality by contact with questioning parents."

It was amongst the infants who required a prolonged period of convalescence, as at the Babies Hospital for infants with tuberculosis and severe rickets, that the observations of the damaging effects of the separation from their parents – the phase of 'Detachment' – were particularly worrying. In

117

the days before effective antibiotic treatment for tuberculosis, these children needed special nursing care and good nourishment in comfortable surroundings for prolonged periods of time, which might not have been available in their homes.

J.C. was well aware of their special needs and although he again did not write explicitly about their emotional needs, he did promote special arrangements for them. From Blagdon Hall in Northumberland, he recorded in the Annual Report of 1943 the special provisions that were made for them, according to their ages, despite the restrictions of the war. He also thought:

"It would be better if the children (in long-stay hospitals) lived in small groups under a house-mother, and from there went to their lessons in a school, to their treatment in a sick bay, and to their entertainment in a central hall. There would be no disadvantage in the house-mother having had a nurse training, but that in itself is not the qualification for the work she will do. Her duty is to live with her group of children and attempt to provide the things of which they have been deprived."[27]

There are other indications that J.C. did indeed understand very well the emotional needs of children, but he openly acknowledged his difficulty in writing about emotions because of unresolved problems of definition. In The Purpose of the Family: a Guide to the Care of Children. 1946,[52] he wrote:

"At one end of the scale emotions come near to reactive feelings, at the other end to acquired sentiment."

Was this perhaps a significant factor in the lack of explicit detailed comment on the psychological aspects of the emotions of children in some of his writings, compounded by his distrust of psychological/psychiatric theories and explanations? He was nevertheless insistent on explaining:

"The view I wish to propound is that as physical health must be developed at each stage by nourishment, play and exercise so it is with emotional health and emotional development," and "The purpose of the family is to give scope for emotional experience."

He went on to describe the needs of children at successive ages and stages of development. In the early years, he comments that at 6-7 months, the individual attention of the mother or of someone who acts as the mother, is necessary:

"If these materials are lacking or if the environment is harmful, the development may be checked, and the loss may never be made good, leaving the child less in stature and sensitivity than it should have been."

For the age of 2 years, he reiterates the need for individual attention from one person or another and records tellingly:

"We must question the methods and results of those public nurseries where too many young children are kept together in a communal life which is imposed on them before they are ready for it."

For the 4 year old, he states:

"The child needs the propinquity of its mother or someone else to whom it may go immediately for reassurances."

He recorded:

"I have had the opportunity to study these effects at close hand at the Babies Hospital."

One of the obituaries written about him records:

"He tried to give every child what he knew his wife would like her children to have."[1]

It is evident that he was writing about the emotional as well as the physical needs of children with a confident and wide knowledge of their needs based on his personal and professional practical experience.

Dr Robertson introduced the account of his studies of 'Separation and the Very Young' as 'A Phase in Paediatric History'. This seems now an appropriate way to explain in part the incongruity of J.C.'s views in relation to the care of children in hospital.

Dr Bowlby had concluded, at the end of his study in 1951, that there was still considerable 'ignorance' about the processes and extent of maternal deprivation despite a quarter of a century of research – precisely the era during which J.C. was actively engaged in the clinical work at the Babies Hospital. A lack of appreciation of psychological principles also applied to many paediatricians in the country.

Dr Bowlby took on board the findings of his colleague, Dr Robertson, after the publication of his report for WHO in 1951. Several papers providing further insights were published during 1952-1954 (quoted in[115]), and further films were made of young children in substitute care. These and further researches culminated in the classic account of 'Attachment and Loss' in 1969, later amplified in 1997[115], in which Bowlby suggested an alternative to the prevailing 'behavioural' theory whereby attachment was held to derive from the provision of nourishment to the child from the mother or other caretaker. Instead, on the basis of extensive experimental studies on children and evidence from observations in the animal world, he proposed what came to be known as an 'evolutionary' theory.[116] Attachment was now held to be the product of a powerful, instinctive psychological process, which promoted strong long-term connections between children and their mothers or caretakers. This includes an adaptive element whereby the chances of survival are increased and children are comforted by the close proximity of the mother or caretaker when confronted with stressful, threatening conditions. These new insights led to a deeper understanding of the process of separation and the prevention and alleviation of the damaging effects on children. J.C. did not have the benefit of a knowledge of these new researches during his lifetime.

The involvement of mothers in the care of their children in hospital was slow to improve due to continued opposition from the health professions, until pressure from the public and media persuaded the Ministry of Health to set up an inquiry in 1957 into 'The welfare of children in hospital'. It recommended in 1959, five years after J.C.'s death:

"Parents should be allowed to visit their sick children whenever they can and to help as much as possible in the care of their child." (The Platt Report)[117]

Opposition continued to such an extent that these recommendations were not mandatory, to be implemented only when the health authorities were ready to do so.

Limited knowledge of underlying psychological mechanisms was not the only consideration that probably played a part in J.C.'s attitude. Although there was during that era a widespread antipathy by physicians towards psychiatrists and psychologists, his outright rejection of the insights of psychology and psychiatry is less easy to explain. It is a matter of speculation, but it seems relevant from a historical perspective to consider some indications amongst his writings that may shine a light on some of the factors that influenced his point of view.

There is one revealing reference of his distrust of Freudian psycho-analytic theory, which informed the practice of psychologists and psychiatrists during the first half of the 20th century.[118a] Commenting on the importance of the mother and child relationship in his lecture on 'The Purpose of the Family'[52] he recorded:

"I would not mention a matter so obvious to you were not the attitudes and sentiments of mothers in danger of being perverted by a cult of too much hygiene which makes them afraid, and by misreadings of Freudian theories which makes them guilty. Under these influences many mothers deny themselves these natural outlets of feelings in contact and companionship with their children, and that leads to an atrophy of maternal function and worse."

Apart from his disdain for psychiatry, he was also averse to bringing social workers into hospitals. He made it clear to Dr Robertson that he considered that the role of the paediatrician included the 'social' care of families. Apart from his rejection of such a multidisciplinary approach, his attitude towards the social sciences also rejected their methods in the investigation of family life:

"It would be churlish of me to leave the impression that the efforts of social scientists have been in vain. I am concerned only to show that their line of country is not across our fields, that the study of the family requires a fresh approach by those trained in the method of the biological sciences, and that in the meantime the practical life of the family is best known through apprenticeship and experience."

120

He goes on to recommend:

"Here I would make a parenthetical claim for two groups of people who are well provided with opportunities for the studies I have suggested. The first group is in danger of extinction. The second is struggling for survival. They are the village schoolmaster and family physician. Both of these can dispose their lives to remain within a community for a generation or more, and so to know it well. They can combine their vocation with an intimacy of social life which is rarely given to those in other vocations."

These comments are consistent with J.C.'s approach to clinical medicine; systematic, empirical observations and practical, pragmatic solutions to the ill health of children in the context of the stages of their development, their families and their environment. His early interest in biochemistry is an indication of his penchant for "the method of the biological sciences." In this context, it is of interest that J.C. also recommended "the scientific method" to attempt the treatment of 'problem families'[18]

His rejection of social workers in a hospital setting in addition to the disciplines of psychology and psychiatry are also in keeping with his all-inclusive view of the role of physicians treating children, before the advent of integrated multidisciplinary systems that include the wider community services. It was not until the early 1970s that a working party of the BPA with the Association of Social Workers would seek a national policy acceptable to both. It was also during those years that the BPA gave a strong voice to the need to recognise and strengthen the professional relationship between paediatrics and child psychiatry. Professor Court, with his extensive experience during J.C.'s 1000 Families Studies in Newcastle, was chairman of the Academic Board of the BPA during 1969-1972 and led the discussions. The publication on behalf of the BPA of 'Paediatrics in the Seventies. Developing the child health services' "was a landmark in stating the criteria and practical conditions for integration of services."[119]

It was well known that J.C. was prone to hyperbole and exaggeration.[8] Like many in the medical profession of his generation, he read widely in the literature of the humanities as well as the sciences and from time to time referred to these in his writings and lectures. A good example follows immediately the comment that has just been recorded in relation to the social sciences:

"Armed with something less than the industry of Gilbert White, or the patience of Charles Darwin over his garden worms, they (that is the schoolmaster and the family doctor) should be able to give us the answer to any of the questions which face us."

Gilbert White was a naturalist like Charles Darwin. They wrote about earthworms, which for J.C. represented a metaphor for 'industry' and 'utility' in a natural setting (see Appendix 5 for details[120 and 121]). J.C. was also fond of poetry, which explains his disconcerting assertion to Dr Robertson of Wordsworth's sometimes unbalanced emotional state as no hindrance to his sublime poetry.

121

His successor, Professor Court was also famously fond of quoting W.H. Auden and T.S. Eliot.

Dr Robertson concluded after his first meeting with J.C. in Newcastle that he had witnessed:

"The idiosyncrasies of one man, his particular fusion of empathy and blindness," only to discover later that "this could also be true of other leading paediatricians."

He went on to record:

"These encounters with Professor Spence and other paediatricians led me to a view about how defences worked throughout the hospital professions in Britain, a view confirmed when I later travelled around the world – how paediatricians could have kind intentions towards children and from these kind intentions had developed areas of considerate practice; yet also have areas of harmful practice to which they were blind because they were not trained in psychological development and because anxieties became repressed in order to sustain a peaceful status quo."

All the evidence from J.C.'s commentaries, publications and keystone lectures suggest that he did have a thorough understanding of child development and empathy for the emotional needs of children and their families. He may not have had a proper understanding and affinity with the psychological processes that operate in maternal deprivation, as far as these were known at the time, but he was one of the first to take practical steps to make use of his knowledge and experience to promote and improve significantly the care of young children in hospital at a time when life threatening conditions dominated the attentions of the health professions. He also wanted to include all mothers in the care of their children on the paediatric wards of the main hospitals; he was against the status quo and did not repress his anxieties. The practical steps that he initiated met the emotional needs of the youngest children under his care at the Babies Hospital, even though he was at pains to emphasise that 'sentiment' did not play any part in the implementation of his proposals. They would also have met, to a large extent, those of all ages admitted to the paediatric wards of the main hospitals during his lifetime, if his recommendations for the accommodation of all mothers had been fulfilled. There is no further documentation of J.C.'s attitude during the remaining years of his life between 1952 and 1954.

There was still much opposition to change amongst the medical profession in the years after his death. In November 1952, Dr Robertson had recorded the immediate angry reaction of paediatricians who saw the premiere of the film, 'A Two-year-old Goes to Hospital', at the Royal Society of Medicine in November 1952. There was a general feeling that they had been slandered. However, at least one paediatrician, Dr Dermod MacCarthy quickly understood the implications and changed the arrangements on his paediatric wards. The circumstances are described in Appendix 6, as an example of what could be achieved very quickly once mothers were welcomed into the hospital to participate in the care of their children.

Dr MacCarthy then promoted his views and practices in a report entitled 'The Emotional Well-being of Children Aged 0-5 Years in Hospital', first published in 1979 by the National Association for the Welfare of Children in Hospital (NAWCH).[122] It was originally requested by The Confederation of European Societies of Paediatricians (of the European Economic Community) and presented to the confederation at a meeting in May 1973. He summarised the "outworn" objections to the admission of mothers with their young children to hospital alongside the "good reasons" (notes in Appendix 6). He comments significantly that the report "generated some heat." It may thus be suggested that the opposition of influential paediatricians nearly two decades after J.C.'s death reinforces the view that his own opposition was not just due to personal "blindness" and "idiosyncrasy" as suggested by Dr Robertson, but was related to a long standing phase in the history of paediatrics during which knowledge of children's emotional development and the effects of maternal deprivation were still deficient. The seminal studies by Bowlby of 'Attachment and Loss' (1969 and 1997[115]) were not published during J.C.'s lifetime. It may also be suggested that his paternalistic approach whereby 'the doctor knows best' combined with his rejection of psychiatry were widely held by the profession.[118b] This was compounded by entrenched practices to suit the requirements and convenience of all the staff and administrators of hospitals and by the lack of an effective 'voice' for parents, which persisted for a long time after the publication of the recommendations of the Platt Report in 1959, which recommended free and frequent access of parents to children's wards.

There may have been some resolution towards the end of J.C.'s life. During the late 1970s, there was a suggestion in Newcastle that he had 'refused' to meet Dr Robertson on a visit to the city. There is no record of the purpose of this visit. More recently, his wife, Joyce Robertson, confirmed that J.C. had kept him waiting in the Children's Clinic at the RVI and then refused to meet him.[123] However, H.S. has a clear recollection that Dr E. Ellis told him that J.C. had "made his peace" with him on a subsequent meeting.

Professor Court, after his succession to the Chair of Child Health in Newcastle in 1955, responded to the new insights about the emotional needs of children and taught the importance of these principles to students and doctors. The film 'A Two-year-old Goes to Hospital' was shown in Newcastle to medical students during their introductory seminars in paediatrics and to nurses and many associated with the care of children in hospital. He was a strong supporter of the establishment of the disciplines of child psychology and psychiatry in Newcastle after 1957.[15] Later, Dr Sydney Bandon, a distinguished psychiatrist born in County Durham and educated at Newcastle University, was invited to participate in the 1000 Families Study and made a significant contribution to the third publication in 1974 about the school years in Newcastle upon Tyne.[40]

Dr Christine Cooper, who had experience of the psycho-analytic aspects of child development under Anna Freud in London and was familiar with the work of Dr Bowlby, Dr Robertson and Dr MacCarthy, also put these insights into

123

practice as early as the 1950s at a residential nursery and later at the Babies Hospital in the1960s and the Fleming Memorial Hospital after 1977.

A letter of appreciation sent to the Platt Inquiry by the mother of a 20 month old child who died from cystic fibrosis after several admissions during the 1950s to the Babies Hospital describes her appreciation of the sensitive care that she received and the benefits to the child and to herself of the opportunity that was available to stay with her and care for her before she died in the hospital. She wrote:

"To have sent her to a ward might not have mattered to her at two-and-a-half months: it would have been cruel at 18 months. She had been ill for 3 months and had had my undivided attention all that time. To have been catapulted from that to loneliness would have been dreadful. As it was, although she fought the treatment every time, and got frightened, I was with her and she had many happy hours right up to the last week."

The legacy that J.C. left of appropriate mother and child accommodation and sensitive care by diligent doctors and nurses was a vital element of the care of this child and her mother. This letter was amongst many sent by parents to the Platt Committee. (Appendix 7, Letter 11[113]).

At the early stages of this study of the legacy of J.C. in February 2015, The Observer newspaper, which had campaigned in the early 1960s for unrestricted visiting of children in hospital, reported a similar campaign for patients at the other end of the age scale, who are afflicted by dementia.[124] Referring to the film 'A Two-year-old Goes to Hospital', it is pointed out:

"At the time, parents were either forbidden to see their children or visit for only an hour a day. One mother wrote of her 20-month-old daughter, hospitalised with an eye infection: "Unable to see, she was taken from me into a strange building full of strange and unfamiliar sounds. She was terrified and bewildered." Substitute the toddler for a 70 year old with dementia, and the unnecessary pain and suffering, in the name of healing, is horrendously similar. It isn't malice at work but bureaucracy and fear of change."

The controversies during J.C.'s lifetime resonate to this day.

The relationship between paediatrics, child psychology and psychiatry in Newcastle developed markedly after the establishment of the Nuffield Psychology and Psychiatry Unit for Children and Young People in 1957 and the appointment of Dr (later Professor) Israel Kolvin in1964. In a notable counterpoint to the attitude of J.C., the amicable and productive collaborations that were developing between paediatrics and psychiatry played an essential part in the service initiated by Dr Cooper for the purposes of child protection, which continued for 43 years following the death of J.C. in 1954. During the 1990s, a number of paediatric registrars were made welcome by Professor Kolvin to participate in training in his department.

The number of children affected and damaged by abuse and neglect was considerable and remains so to this day. Many, including newborn babies are still at risk of significant harm at the hands of their parents and caretakers. At the time of conducting this study in 2014, there emerged a report about the work of the English Family courts over a seven year period from 2007 to 2013. 7,143 birth mothers appeared in 15,645 recurrent care proceedings concerning no less than 22,790 infants and children.[126]

Although participation in help for children with suspected child sexual abuse was undertaken only in a very small number of children on a residential basis, it has been given prominence because this form of abuse did not come to the fore until 1986 in Newcastle, long after other forms of abuse had been widely recognised. The high prevalence in the childhood population had hitherto not been appreciated in Newcastle; and the northern districts, as elsewhere in the United Kingdom, by the medical services; even very young children seemed to have been at risk in large numbers.[125] It required an urgent response from paediatricians whose knowledge of the nature and diagnosis was very limited. The condition had not been recorded in the admissions to the Babies Hospitals and J.C. and his colleagues made no mention of it. Only Dr Cooper and later a handful of doctors from the Northumbria Women Police Doctors Scheme had any expertise. It was a watershed for paediatrics and a call for a better understanding and recognition of the problem. The legacy of J.C.'s insights into the importance of family, environmental and social factors for the health and welfare of children were of fundamental importance to the development of paediatric services for these children and families. Child psychiatry services under the direction of Professor Kolvin played an important part in the assessments of the families that took place during that time.

At the Newcastle hospital facilities only a handful of rooms were ever available for the assessment and support of 'problem families'. Nevertheless, during a period of 14 years from March 1977 to 1 April 1991, 650 children were admitted for help and support of their parents and caretakers and in many cases for an assessment of their ability to care for them safely and appropriately.[14] These were in the main young children under the age of 3 years with a majority under the age of 1 year.

The six surveys of outcome during 1978 to 1994 reveal that a majority of the children admitted to the special hospital facilities with their parents or caretakers went home immediately after a residential assessment, but a significant and increasing proportion went into foster care after the breakdown of their care at home. Nevertheless, it was evident that in these very vulnerable families in which there were serious risks of harm and neglect to their children, nearly half (46%) of the children were still at home in 1996, two to four years after discharge from the Family Unit. One of the children placed later in foster care had sustained a further fracture, but to the best of our knowledge none of the others were seriously harmed or neglected in their homes as their families were closely supervised and social services intervened when their care was no longer satisfactory or safe. In earlier years before the availability of such a residential assessment and less well developed community services, it is likely that many of these children, especially the newborn babies at risk, would not have been allowed home or rehabilitated to the care of their parents or caretakers

It is noteworthy that many families (about 30%) admitted to the Family Unit in 1992-1994 had further children two to four years after the completion of their residential assessment. This applied equally to those whose children went into foster care as in those allowed home. It raises the possibility of an increased risk of harm to their health and welfare because of 'continuities of deprivation'.

The consequences of childhood deprivations were investigated in Newcastle in 300 families from the 1000 Families Study.[41] By 1979-80, when these children had reached the age of 32-33 years, seven main types of deprivation were identified: marital disruption, parental illness, poor domestic care of the child and the home, dependence on social services, overcrowding, poor mothering and educational disability. It was found that the greatest risk of harm to the children occurred in the group of families with multiple deprivations coexisting in the same families. The extent of a 'continuity of deprivation' was of the order of 50%.

These were precisely the types of risk that were often identified in various combinations during the assessments at the Mother and Child and Family Units in Newcastle during 1977-1997 in the families who had harmed their children or were considered to be at severe risk of doing so. The study of the 300 children from 1000 Families did not directly address the risks of child abuse amongst them; the number was too small for this purpose. There is just one reference to physical abuse in the children who had accidents that required medical attention, which were much more common in families with multiple deprivations (58%) than in those who were not deprived (26%). It was suggested:

"Since in the deprived group a relative absence of accidents proved to be associated with resilience, it is reasonable to speculate that, in the multiply deprived group, accidents represent a combination of carelessness and ineffective care or perhaps even physical abuse."

It was evident however, that "individuals vary in their resilience to environmental experiences and that different undesirable experiences may have different risk potentials" for harm, especially in the areas of cognitive, social, emotional and behavioural development. It is reasonable to add child abuse and neglect to this list of potential harmful consequences. It was also recorded that "our work emphasises the importance of a network of social and emotional support, especially in the pre-school years, as protection against environmental deprivation."

An important new insight also emerged during the early 1980s, that Bowlby in his studies of maternal deprivation had probably overestimated the 'universality' and 'irreversibility' of psychological consequences.[127 and 128] It follows that all these considerations are very likely to apply to child abuse and neglect. They provide evidence for the validity of the opportunities to allow some of the most vulnerable 'problem families' to continue to care for children that they had harmed and neglected or were at severe risk of doing so. This was notwithstanding all the risks and considerable resources required for assessment, support, practical help and treatment, often on a long term basis. There was also an awareness that fostering and adoption were, in some cases, beset with problems with harm to the children. Although overwhelmingly worthwhile, they are not always successful.[129]

Although the 'cycle of deprivation' - a phrase made famous in a speech by Sir Keith Joseph in 1972, then Secretary of State for Social Services, at a conference for local authorities organised by the Pre-school Playgroup Association[130] – was evident in many families whose children required protection, it was:

"Intended to apply to families in the greatest adversity and was not necessarily thought to have direct implications for parent-child resemblance across the social spectrum."

There was no association of abuse and neglect with multiple deprivations in some families who were assessed in the residential hospital facilities in Newcastle during the two decades after 1977. For example, poor tolerance to the day-to-day stresses of life or 'immaturity' of young single parents without adequate knowledge of child care were the predominant risks in some families. The collaboration between paediatrics, child psychology and psychiatry in the residential assessment of these vulnerable families ensured a more secure understanding of the problems of these families.

During this period, as far as it was known, the Mother and Child Unit at the Fleming Hospital and the Family Unit at Newcastle General Hospital were the only paediatric hospital residential resources nationwide that undertook this work with such young children from vulnerable 'problem families'. There was one other Family Unit in Britain, located in a children's psychiatric hospital at Oxford, with a close paediatric involvement.[131] The consultant paediatrician there, Dr Margaret Lynch, had been a junior doctor in Dr Cooper's Department in Newcastle. That service at the Park Hospital for Children in Oxford, in contrast to the Family Unit in Newcastle, dealt with children with a variety of psychological and psychiatric disorders in addition to child abuse and neglect. They also undertook psychotherapy for the family dysfunctions that underlie these problems. In Newcastle, appropriate psychotherapy was available for only a few families after the period of residential assessment alongside support, help and supervision by the community health, social services or NSPPC in the community.

In the end, the demise of the Family Unit in 1997, the last descendant of the Babies Hospital, and the transfer of this service into the community may also be linked to elements of J.C.'s legacy. He and his colleagues had already indicated four decades earlier in the 1000 Families Study that community workers, "may play a larger part" in the support of 'problem families'.[18] The product of all the community studies that followed eventually played a significant part in the emergence of a new branch of paediatrics – 'community' or 'social paediatrics'- which led to a diminishing reliance in Newcastle and the northern districts on hospital paediatric services for the assessment and support of 'problem families', but also on the active involvement of paediatricians, not just as 'field workers' from the hospitals, but as consultants in the community child health services. In 2001, the need for paediatricians to work in close collaboration with all those concerned with child protection was upheld in order to provide the most appropriate service and maintain the confidence to work in such a stressful area of paediatrics.[132]

There was one other residential resource in Newcastle, the Ryehill Family Centre under the aegis of the Social Services Department, which also closed (in 1993) mainly due to financial constraints.

The data that is still accessible about the clinical work of the West End Day Nursery, the Babies Hospitals at West Parade, Blagdon Hall and Leazes Terrace, and their descendants at the Fleming Memorial and Newcastle General Hospitals, is incomplete in certain aspects and allowances have been made accordingly. This is not surprising in a retrospective survey of archives over this length of time. Nevertheless, the information and commentaries that are available allow for the description of the essential contents and stages in the development of the special services that are a basis for this assessment of J.C.'s legacy.

The inclusion of a detailed account of the nature of the activities and outcome in relation to child protection is intended to demonstrate that J.C.'s legacy is manifest even in those areas of paediatrics, which had not yet come to the fore during his lifetime. The priorities that arose in later years required the application of his principal insights about the appropriate hospital care of sick babies and infants, the attention to the needs of their mothers and especially the realisation of the vital contribution of social-environmental factors to the health, development and welfare of children and their families.

The records of the finances in the Annual Reports of the Babies Hospital (Appendix 3) provide an insight into the considerable efforts that were made to sustain and develop the services of the hospital before the advent of the National Health Service. J.C. played a leading part as chairman of the medical staff and a member of the Management Committee. Although the accounts were always in balance - expenditure was always equal to income - an overdraft had to be sought from the banks during most of the life of the hospital. It was readily granted and it was only in 1945 that this was cleared, mainly due to the largest recorded legacy during that final year.

From the outset in 1926, two decades before the advent of the NHS in 1948, extensive public funds were already granted by the Ministry of Health and the councils of Newcastle upon Tyne and the northern districts. These amounted to over 40% of income during the 1930s and over 50% during the years of the Second World War. The numerous private donations and subscriptions, amounting to a high of a third of the income during 1940-1944, were an essential contribution. Although about a third of the largest donations (£50 and over) came from less than 2% of donors, the records show that the great majority gave relatively small amounts - an average of £4. The earnings of the majority of working families were insufficient to pay for the inpatient pay treatment of their children. The private fees from mothers contributed only about 6% of the income up to 1944.

The successful, albeit difficult, balance of the accounts was achieved ultimately by the recognition of the excellence of the clinical service, available to all in Newcastle and the northern districts and further afield. Right from the outset, J.C. provided the inspiration and leadership that ensured the friendly collaboration between all the professional, public and private interests that were involved.

The contribution of the Babies Hospital and its descendants is only one element of J.C.'s legacy. There remain his promotion of the education of students, doctors, administrators and the public in the diseases of childhood, his influence on local and national policies concerning service provision and research, and his masterful ability to communicate the significant components of paediatric knowledge and the means that are necessary for the treatment and care of children and their families. The unique importance of the Babies Hospital is that it provided him with a clinical platform to develop the ideas and practices that inspired future generations concerned with the health and welfare of children and their families. It was eventually also a launch pad for the specialist hospital service that evolved in order to participate in the multidisciplinary activities related to child protection during the later part of the 20th century.

The 1000 Family Study that he initiated continues to this day to provide evidence of the contribution of socioeconomic conditions and life styles to the wellbeing of the population. It also contributes to a greater understanding of the medical, educational, social and economic policies that may contribute most to a healthier and more fulfilling life for children and their families.

During this narrative, three colleagues, appointed and encouraged by J.C., emerge as leading proponents of his legacy. Dr Fred Miller was responsible for the initial practical work associated with the Thousand Families Study and contributed to further researches in later childhood. Dr Donald Court, who succeeded him as the first James Spence Professor of Child Health, also began his contribution in this study. During the 3000 home visits that he undertook during a period of 15 years:

"The insights gained from these visits profoundly influenced his perspective throughout his professional life; for him, the child was never seen in isolation but always as part of a family, which in turn was part of a neighbourhood and the wider community." [133]

He went on to promote the education of medical students by taking a leading part in the introduction in 1962 of a new curriculum at the university in tune with modern requirements.[101a] He also supported the development of sub-specialisation in Newcastle in response to the imperatives of new knowledge and the fruitful collaboration with Child Psychology and Psychiatry and the Speech Department of the University. During the years of his retirement, he led the profession towards an integration of all the national services for children and their families. Dr Christine Cooper was inspired by J.C.'s empathic approach to children and families. She took on the task of protecting children from harm and neglect and supporting vulnerable families when this became a priority for paediatricians a decade after his death. In the process, she went a step further than J.C. by taking on board the multidisciplinary activities with social workers, psychologists and psychiatrists that came to be an essential part of the prevention and management of these conditions.

129

The authors of this study are some of the beneficiaries of J.C.'s legacy. They trained in Newcastle and went on to pursue lifelong careers in Tyneside.

The special interest of the Newcastle University Department of Child Health in the community and social aspects of Paediatrics and Child Health initiated by the researches and teaching of J.C. and his colleagues was strengthened further by the establishment of the Donald Court Chair of Community Child Health in 1993. The initiative came from Sir Liam Donaldson, the contemporary Regional Medical Officer of Health, influenced by Professor Court's Report to the Secretaries of State for England and Wales – "Fit for the Future. The Report of the Committee on Child Health Services", 1976, which Professor Court chaired.

The culture of friendship and respectful collaboration between all those associated with the care of children and a special interest in social paediatrics in the Department of Child Health in Newcastle are some of the most distinctive elements of his legacy. Dr Ellis drew attention also to J.C.'s remarks to him:

"My job is to provide the conditions in which you can do good work".[8]

The picture that emerges of Sir James Spence's involvement in the West End Nursery and the Babies Hospital in Newcastle upon Tyne enhances significantly an understanding of the origins and evolution of his legacy. The life of the special hospital units that followed also provides a new insight into the contribution of the legacy to the response to priorities, notably the maltreatment and neglect of children, which came later to the fore in paediatrics.

Most of his ideas have stood the test of time. The ones that did not were in many ways a reflection of the ethos of an era when a paternalistic approach by physicians was common and paediatrics and child health were being established as new specialities in medicine. Subspecialities, multidisciplinary practices and an effective 'voice' for parents had not yet evolved sufficiently to have an influence on the delivery of health services to hospitals and the community.

His achievements and inspiration, however, had a profound impact for good on the health and welfare of children and their families and the development of paediatrics in Newcastle, the northern districts and nationwide.

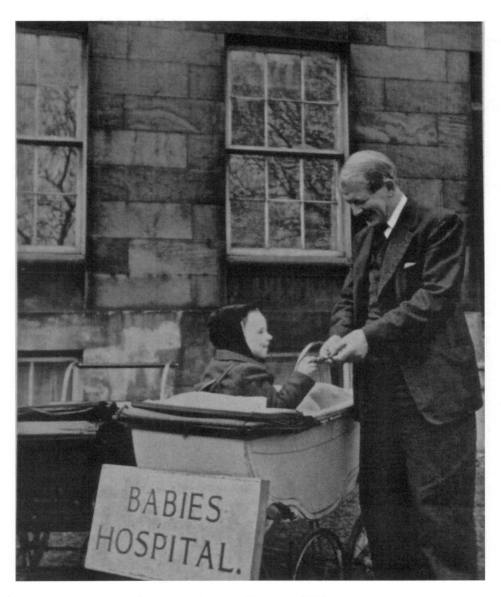

Professor Sir James Spence at Leazes Terrace, 1953
From Lady Ridley's Memoir

APPENDICES

Appendix 1. Tables

Table 1: The Babies Hospital and Mothercraft Centre at West Parade. 1925-1936

	1925-26*	1926	1927	1928	1929	1930	1931	1932	1933	1934	1935	1936
Number of beds	17	17	17	17	17	17	22	22	26	26	36	36
Rooms for mother and child	1	1	1	2	2	2	8	8	8	8	8	8
Number of new inpatients	86	102	106	115	186	213	222	275	308	310	321	339
Total number in hospital	98	119	123	133	202	229	243	291	326	329	342	355
Number of resident mothers	9	9	11	8	7	17	28	45	41	29		70
- % of new admissions	11%	9%	10%	7%	4%	8%	13%	16%	13%	9%		21%
Average length of stay (days)		41	44		29			21	21	24	27	19
Outcome on discharge:												
- total number		81	89		134	168	171	207	247	243	223	252
- % cured		72	61		54	57	88	88	51	53	47	48
- % improved		13	29		40	42	-	12	14	41	44	39
- % iSQ or transferred		15	10		6	1	12	-	35	6	9	13
Died	12	21	17		36	49	48	63	61	67	60	69
- Percent of all inpatients	12%	18%	14%		18%	21%	20%	22%	19%	20%	18%	19%
Outpatients:												
- new referrals									663	811	685	911
- total number		143	427	877	1409	1004	755		2285	2451	2101	?

Age on admission	Average per year (%)	Range (%)
Up to 3 months	38	27-53
Over 3-6 months	16	12-22
Over 6-12 months	18	12-24
Over 12 months	28	22-39

Table 2: The Babies Hospital and Mothercraft Centre at West Parade.1925-1936

Principal diseases and disorders treated at the hospital

	1925 to 1926	1926	1927	1928	1929	1930	1931	1932	1933	1934	1935	1936
Re-establishment and maintenance of breastfeeding	5	9	6	8	5							
Feeding difficulties											14	32
Marasmus	43	55	34	19	32	12	13					
Dyspepsia		9							27	19	18	14
Rickets		7	4	10	25	26	11	22	17	10	11	
Infections Percent of all admissions		7 (7%)	10 (9%)	18 (16%)	35 (19%)	63 (30%)	60 (27%)	70 (25%)	123 (40%)	109 (35%)	95 (30%)	103 (30%)
Infective enteritis		7	5	14	14	15		17	36	40	15	43
General sepsis and its effects						20	22	25	43	10	37	46
Paratyphoid fever						2						
Lung infections			5		21	21	38	24	36	52	38	14
Meningitis				4		3		4	8	7	5	
Acute anterior polio						2						
Tuberculosis	10		7	7	15	17	16	20	11	11	16	15
Chronic chest disorders				10	2	6						4
Gastro-intestinal disorders			10	1			18					
Prematurity and newborn disorders		4	3		9	10		7			10	13
Congenital disorders	4		8	5	3	7		24	45	49	59	13
Hare lip and cleft palate												55 *
Pyloric stenosis	6	8	12	12	14	22	15	40	23	33	37	27
Anaemia					4	5	9				6	8
Diabetes					1							
Coeliac disease		1	2		2			5				
Pink Disease		2		6	5	9	14	10	5	5	4	6
Skin disease			3		9							
Kidney disease				9	12	7						
Miscellaneous medical conditions	18		7	10	13	29						

* Includes hare lip 26 and cleft palate 29

134

Table 3a: Sources of Referral. Babies Hospital at West Parade. 1926-1939

	1926	1927	1928	1929	1930	1931	1932	1933	1934	1935	1936	1937	1938	1939
Newcastle	43	44	51	82	101	131	122	129	122	128	127	127	87	73
%	53%	47%	54%	44%	47%	59%	47%	43%	40%	43%	37%	35%	25%	24%
Northumberland	5	10	16	22	20	21	28	26	28	31	36	41	85	69
Durham	21	14	18	26	21	29	31	50	60	55	51	70	94	93
Gateshead		4	11	20	22	9	22	36	30	18	24	30	29	32
Other northern districts		9	13	36	49	32	52	57	70	63	95	70	32	25
Yorkshire							1					4		
Glasgow							1							
Rugby										1				
Potters Bar										1				
Derby											1			
Preston											1			
Other hospitals	12	12	6									20	27	15
Private practice practitioners	21	12					18	10	6	24				
NSPCC		1												
Total	102	106	115	186	213	222	275	308	310	321	339	358	354	307

Table 3b: Sources of Referral. Babies Hospital at Blagdon Hall. 1940-44

Table 3b   Sources of Referral. Babies Hospital at Blagdon Hall. 1940-44

	1940	1941	1942	1943	1944
Newcastle	39 17%	40 18%	36 14%	54 22%	33 18%
Northumberland	56	30	58	27	17
Durham	61	66	69	64	66
Gateshead	30	20	25	19	8
Other northern districts	40	53	64	72	57
Yorkshire	4	6	7	7	1
Lincolnshire	2	1			
Derbyshire	2				1
Scotland	2	1	1		
Cheshire		1			
Kent		1			
Hampshire			1		
Buckinghamshire					1
Coventry					1
Total	236	219	261	243	186

135

Table 4: The Babies Hospital. 1937-1945
At West Parade, Newcastle, 1937 to 31 August 1939, then at Blagdon Hall, Northumberland, 1 September 1939 - 1945

	1937	1938	1939	1940	1941	1942	1943	1944	1945 (1)
New inpatients	358	354	307	236	219	261	243	186	
Total number in hospital	376			247	230	281	264		58
Number of resident mothers (2)	71	104	89	85	67	94	87	70	
- Percent of new admissions	20%	29%	29%	36%	31%	36%	36%	38%	
Length of stay (average; days)	16	15	15	16	17	23			
Operations					92		106	82	
Outcome on discharge									
- total number		290	274	208	181	220	200		58
- % cured		86	55	59	77	66	74		31
- % improved, ISQ or transferred		-	32	28	14	23	20		57
		14	13	13	9	11	6		12
Died		64	33	17	27	20	22	NONE	NONE
- Percent of new admissions		18%	11%	7%	12%	8%	9%		
Outpatients									
- new referrals	998	1068		801	712	715	1644	1642	
- total number				2049	1734	1544	3571	3569	

Age on admission	Average per year (%)	Range (%)	1945. Convalescents at Blagdon Hall	
- up to 4 months	50	49-54	Under 1 month	5
			1-2 years	19
- 4-6 months	12	11-14	2-5 years	28
- 7-12 months	29	24-36	5-8 years	6
- Over 12 months	9	6-14		

1. In 1945, admissions were restricted to convalescent children
2. From 1940 to 1944, at Blagdon Hall, there was still accommodation for 36 children and 8 resident mothers

Table 5a: Discrepancies in the recording of data relating to the total number of admissions and diagnoses and the separate identification of hare lip and cleft palate during 1929 to 1939

	1929	1930	1931	1932	1933	1934	1935	1936	1937	1938	1939
Total number of admissions	186	213	222	275	308	310	321	339	358	354	307
Total number of diagnoses	186	213	156	198	251	236	243	282	357	347	306
Shortfall	-	-	-66 30%	-77 28%	-57 19%	-74 24%	-78 24%	-57 17%	1 0.2%	10 3%	1 0.3%

Table 5b: The recording of congenital malformations including hare lip and cleft palate between 1929 and 1935 and the separate recording of hare lip and cleft palate between 1936 and 1939 [1]

	1929	1930	1931	1932	1933	1934	1935	1936	1937	1938	1939
Total number of congenital malformations including hare lip and cleft palate [2]	3	7	-	24	45	49	59	13	23	4	2
Separate recording of hare lip and cleft palate	-	-	-	-	-	-	-	55	38	38	63

1. The first operation (for hare lip) was recorded in 1929
2. Separate recording of these two categories continued after 1939 (Table 7)

137

Table 6: The Babies Hospital. 1937-1945
Medical diseases and disorders treated at the hospital

	1937	1938	1939	1940	1941	1942	1943	1944	1945
Feeding difficulties	48	46	34	23	19	23	17	12	
Malnutrition				3	6	7	10	2	5
Dyspepsia				4	1		2		
Rickets			4	2	3	2	2		
Scurvy			1						
Infections									
Total number	115	110	74	29	41	37	43	30	15
Percent of all	32%	31%	24%	12%	19%	14%	18%	16%	26%
admissions	28	22	21	10	7	12	15	6	4
Respiratory tract	4	19	5	5	1		7	2	10
Chronic lung				3	10	8		8	
infections	31	28	12	1	1	6	9	4	
Neonatal sepsis	8	10	4	3	6	2	1	1	
Gastroenteritis and			9	2	2	1	5	1	
Dysentery	44	31	2	2					
Meningitis			4	2	3	4	1	3	
Skin sepsis			17	4	11	4	5	5	1
Sepsis and its effect									
Infections of unknown type									
Tuberculosis	33	22	13	13	11	9	17	21	22
Alimentary diseases:	2	5	2	1	1		1		
Intussusception		3	4	1		3	2	1	2
Coeliac disease			9	15	6	12	13	9	2
Nervous diseases			5	1		4	3	1	2
Functional disorders				5	2	1			
Behaviour problems							4	1	
Kidney diseases	3	19	2	2	1	1			
Blood diseases	8	4	3	3	3	1	1	1	
New growths			1	1		6	7	6	2
Skin diseases:									
Eczema	5			4	7	2	2		
Naevus				1			3	1	
Diseases of newborn	15	11	14	3	2	8	4	2	
Traumatic conditions						5	1	2	
Cretinism						1			
Asthma						1			
Pink Disease	7	9	15	5	4	6	3	2	
Miscellaneous medical conditions	21	37	14	8	9	11	9	13	8

Table 7: The Babies Hospital. 1937-1944
Surgical conditions

	1937	1938	1939	1940	1941	1942	1943	1944	1945
Pyloric stenosis	39	39	47	54	35	54	43	33	None
Congenital defects		4	1	2	2	1	1	2	
Hare lip and cleft palate	38	38	63	58	62	60	58	42	
Miscellaneous		6			3			9	

Table 8: The Babies Hospital. 1937-1945
Some details to illustrate the increase in the variety of diagnoses and the various forms of tuberculosis

Infections	Whooping cough 6; thrush 2; otitis media 4; cervical adenitis 6; osteitis 2; stomatitis 2; One each of tapeworm; arthritis; round worm; post-circumcision sepsis; abscess; infective hepatitis; otorhoea; conjunctivitis; congenital syphilis.
Alimentary diseases	pylorospasm 33; peptic ulcer 1; rumination 4; intestinal dysfunction 8; megacolon 1; fissure in ano 1; hernia 6.
Nervous diseases	mental deficiency 6; mongolism 3; hydrocephalus 1; convulsions 5; cerebral tumour 1.
Kidney diseases	Brights disease 8; kidney tumour 1; retention of urine1 .
Blood diseases	anaemia 12; leukaemia 3
New growths	One each of suprarenal tumour; cerebellar tumour; mediastinal tumour; tumour of tongue; lipoma new growths and cysts 6.
Traumatic conditions	cerebral birth trauma 4; burns 2; safety pin in stomach 1; fractured skull 1
Cretinism	1
Scurvy	1
Tuberculosis	Generalised 1 Pulmonary 138 Abdominal 11 Meningitis 8 Adenitis 3 Mastoiditis 1

Table 9: Pyloric stenosis, hare lip and cleft palate at the Babies Hospital.
1929-1944

	1929 - 1935	1936 - 1944
Total number of inpatients	1835	2503
Number of pyloric stenosis (a)	184	371
Number of hare lip and cleft palate (b)	197	476
Total (a) and (b)	371	847
Operations - Percent of all admissions	20%	34%

Record of Operations – includes 'Others' for comparison?

	Total	Pyloric Stenosis	Hare Lip	Cleft Palate	Others
1936			26 (1 died)	21 (1 died)	
1937		36 (3 died)			
1938	80	36 (3 died)	22	16 (1 died)	3 Intussusception 3 Miscellaneous
1940		48	44		
1941	93	34 (3 died)	53 (1 died)		1 each: Excision of burn scar, Pylorospasm and Intussusception, 2 Hernias
1943		39	39		
1944	82	33 (1 died)	21	19	2 Pylorospasm 1 Intestinal dysfunction (died) 6 Removal of tumours and cysts

Table 10: Admissions to the Babies Hospital, Leazes Terrace. 1950-1976

	1950	1955	First 6 months (1 Jan to 30 June) 1960	1965	First 6 months (1 Jan to 30 June) 1973	Up to November 1976
Number of cots	24	24	26	26	26	26
Rooms for mothers	11	11	11	11	11	9
Admitted with mother - % of all admissions		281 60%		319 44%		129 70%
Acute infections	105 (36%)	153 (32%)	36 (13%)	30 (4%)	77 (22%) [1]	25 (14%)
Tuberculosis	23	8	1	1	-	-
Failure to thrive, endocrine and metabolic problems	16	43	12	18	15	36
Feeding difficulties	10	-	5	23	2	4
Congenital heart disease [2]	-	16	17	47	48	-
Other congenital malformations	12	47	11	-	13	-
Neonatal disorders	29	65	24	31	12	-
CNS and developmental problems	8	24	13	38	13 [3]	38
Problems of management and behaviour disorders	16	26	12	13	-	13
Miscellaneous medical conditions	63 [4]	79	69	43	65	23
Social Problem - associated with medical condition - poor care - abuse and neglect - Assessment for adoption	2	-	2 2	-	-	37 (20%) 17 12 8 }11%
Surgical admissions	5 (2%)	17 (4%)	73 (27%)	476 (66%)	103 (30%)	8 (0.4%)
Hernia	-		39		11	
Tracheo-oesophogeal	-				15	
Hirshsprung Disease	-				3	
Diaphragmatic hernia	-				2	
Pyloric stenosis	3				4	
Other	2		34		68	
Total medical admissions	280	461	202	244	245	176
Total admissions	289	478	275	720	348	184
Deaths	20 (7%)		14 (5%)		2 (0.6%)	NONE

1. Includes 35 infants with bronchiolitis (Respiratory Syncitial Virus isolated); 14% of all medical admissions during the first 6 months of that year
2. After 1973, congenital heart disease was investigated and treated at Freeman Hospital in Newcastle
3. Includes 5 children with febrile convulsions (Influenza A virus) compared with only 1 in 1960
4. Includes 7 infants with Pink Disease.

Table 11: Survey of all admissions of children under the age of 12 years admitted to Newcastle hospitals and nursing homes.1943-1944 [27]

Total population in Newcastle	Estimated 260,000
Total number of children under 12 years	Estimated 50,000
Average number of admissions per year	3743 (7.5%)
Trauma – total	306 (8%)
- serious burns and scalds	55
- fractures	77
- head and other serious injuries	56
Acute lung infections – total	312
- pneumonia	150
Abscesses, cellulitis and skin sepsis	202
Tuberculosis – total	129
- tuberculous meningitis or miliary disease	26
- bone	3
Emergency surgery – total	79
- aged under 3 years	31
- appendicitis	42
Planned surgery – total	115
- hernia	60
- orthopaedic operations	23
Specific fevers – total	929 (25%)
- scarlet fever	190
- diphtheria	144
Acute infective enteritis	122
Dysentery	90
Meningococcal meningitis	22
Rheumatic heart disease	15
Venereal disease	7
Nephritis	11
Coeliac disease	7
Total number of principal diseases recorded	2346
Tonsillectomy	
- average number of admissions per year	890
- percent of all the average number of admissions per year	Approximately 24%
Note: Infections comprised 77% of all recorded principal diseases	

142

Table 12: Admissions to the Babies Hospital at Leazes Terrace. 1955

Total number	478
Age	
- Under 1 year	322 (67%)
- Over 1 year	126 (33%)
Mothers admitted	281 (59%)
Sources of referral	
- Family doctor or other hospital	164 (34%)
- From Outpatient Children's Clinic or other hospital department	314 (66%)
Infections	
- Pneumonia and Bronchitis	58
- Meningitis	13
- Urinary infections	14
- Osteitis	21
- Tuberculosis	8
- Other	47
Neonatal Disease	
- Haemolytic disease of newborn (HDN)	18
- Haemorrhagic disease	8
- Birth injury	9
- Prematurity	15
- Others	15
Congenital malformations	
- Congenital heart disease	16
- Urinary tract malformation	9
- Other malformations	38
Failure to thrive	43
Behaviour disorders (problems of management)	26
Obscure and rare diseases	19
Surgical cases	
Hernias	10
Others	7
Mental Deficiency and Spasticity	15
Blood Diseases other than leukaemia and HDN	10
Convulsive disorders	9
Malignant disease (including leukaemia)	7
Miscellaneous (not separately classified)	43

Table 13: Admissions to the Mother and Child Unit at the Fleming Hospital (1978 to October 1987) and the Family Unit Newcastle General Hospital. 1988 to 1 April 1991

	Mother & Child Unit FMH				Family Unit, NGH			
	1978	1983	1985	Up to Oct 1987	1988	1989	1990 (1)	Up to April 1991
Number of cots	7	7	7	7	7	7	7	7
Rooms for mothers	7	7	7	7	5	5	5	5
Total number of admissions	157	152	157	95	96	92	77	22
Admitted with mother		70	73	64	59	53	52	18
- Percent of all admissions [2]		50%	64%	96%	97%	79%	100%	95%
Infections	-	-	8	-	-	-	-	-
Tuberculosis	-	-	-	-	-	-	-	-
Failure to thrive, endocrine and metabolic disorders	-	-	4	-	-	-	-	-
Feeding difficulties	-	-	-	-	-	-	-	
Congenital malformations	-	-	1	-	-	-	-	-
Neonatal disorders	10	12						
CNS and developmental problems	-	-	14	-	-	1		-
Miscellaneous medical conditions	36	39	15	5	2	-	-	-
Problems of management and behaviour disorders	-	-	3	-	-	3	-	1
Social problems - total	76	69	63	62	59	63	52	18
- Associated with medical conditions	24	22	16	12	16	7	20	1
- Issues of child protection	52	47	47	50	43	56	32	17
- poor care			14		16	35	13	10
- child abuse and neglect			20		9	9	7	1
- sexual abuse			1		3	-	1	1
- newborns 'at risk'			12		15	12	11	5
- percent of all admissions	35%	34%	41%	75%	70%	84%	62%	89%
Severe physical and mental disabilities for family relief	10	13	30	16	23	25	25	3
Weekend lodgers from child psychiatry			13	12	12			
Total medical admissions	122	120	108	67	2	4	-	1
Total surgical admissions	25	19	6	-	-	-	-	-
Percentage of admissions with social problems [2]	52%	50%	55%	93%	97%	94%	100%	95%

1. Closed for six weeks due to staff shortages
2. Excludes children with physical and mental disabilites and weekend lodgers

144

Table 14a: Admissions to the Mother and Child Unit, Fleming Hospital. 1985 *

Total number – 144				
Admitted with mother, father, or both parents – 73 (45.6%)				
Additional weekend admissions only from the Nuffield Child Psychiatry Unit - 13				
	Total	**Medical & surgical problems**	**Severe disabilities**	**Medical – social problems**	**Issues of child protection**
---	---	---	---	---	---
Age on admission					
- Up to 1 month	51 (35%)	13	-	11	27
- Over 1-12 months	26 (18%)	11	3	2	10
- Over 1 – 3 years	67 (47%)	27	27	3	10
Over 3 years	NONE	NONE	NONE	NONE	NONE
Admissions					
- With mother	73* (62%)	27	-	11	27
- With father				3	-
- With both parents					5
Sources of Referral					
Newcastle	59 (40%)	15	14	7	23
Northumberland	54	27	13	4	10
Durham	11	4	-	2	5
North Tyneside	9	1	3	4	1
Other northern districts	14	4	-	2	8
Average length of stay (in days)		Less than 7	4	10	21-28

* Excludes children for family relief and the weekend lodgers from the Child Psychiatry Services

Table 14b: Admissions to the Mother and Child Unit. Fleming Hospital.1985 Medical and surgical conditions. Social problems

Medical conditions	Constipation - 8 Convulsions - 6 Failure to thrive - 4 Respiratory infections - 4 Gastroenteritis - 3 Enuresis - 3 Choking attacks in severely physically disabled child - 2 Diabetes - 2 Chest pains following operation for congenital cyst - 2 Behaviour disorders - 3 One each (total 8) of: asthma, hiatus hernia, migraine, obesity (for slimming), developmental delay, depression, oro-facial digital syndrome, recurrent urinary tract infections
Surgical problems (all post-operative)	One each (total 6) of: spina bifida, neonatal intestinal obstruction, choanal-atresia, ischio-rectal abscess, ileostomy following enterocolitis, diaphragmatic hernia
Severe physical and mental disabilities for family relief	30 (6 children)
Admissions from Child Psychiatry Unit at weekends	13
Medical conditions with social problems	Infected eczema / impetigo - 6 Developmental delay - 2 Sleep problems - 2 (twins) One each (total 6) of: post-op exomphalos medical problems, gastroenteritis, incontinence following anal surgery, retention constipation with behavioural problems, Pierre Robin syndrome, failure to thrive associated with enteritis.
Social problems with issues of child protection - Physical abuse - Sexual abuse - Neglect - failure to thrive - Newborn babies 'at risk' - Problems of care in association with varying degrees of family dysfunction, psychiatric illness, chaos and strife	47 13 1 7 10 (2 with siblings) 14

146

Table 15: Assessment and help for 64 children from 49 families with social problems and issues of child protection at the Mother and and Child Unit, Fleming Memorial Hospital. 1984-85

	Total	Discharged home	To foster care	
			After assessment	Later from home
Total number of children	64	49 (77%)	15	5 (10%)*
Newborn babies 'at risk'	25	21 (84%)	4	4 (19%)
Abused and neglected	16	10 (63%)	6	-
Multiple family problems	16	13 (81%)	3	1
Siblings	7	5	2	-
Legal Orders				
Total number (excluding siblings)	21 (37%)			
Home on Court Order: - Newborns 'at risk"	4 (19%) out of 21; 1 to foster care later			
- Abused and neglected	5 (50%) out of 10; 1 to foster care later			

*44 (69%) out of the original 64 children admitted were still at home after an average of one year after discharge from the Mother and Child Unit

Table 16: Admissions to the Family Unit (Newcastle General Hospital) of children from families with social problems and issues of child protection, only for observation, support and treatment. 1988 – 1 April 1991

Total number of families	24
Total number of children, including siblings	31
Admitted with mother	16
mother and father	3
child only	2
parent(s) with siblings	10
Length of stay	
Up to 7 days	20
Over 1 to 3 weeks	7
Over 3 to 6 weeks	3
Over 6 weeks	1
Age of children	
Up to 1 month	4
Over 1 to 12 months	12
Over 1 to 5 years	10
Over 5 to 10 years	3
Over 10 years	2

148

Table 17: Admissions to the Family Unit, Newcastle General Hospital.
Assessment of families with issues of child protection.
1988 to 1 April 1991

	1988	1989	1990	1991 (Jan to 1 April)
Total number of families	34	34	25	13
Total number of children [1]	36	39	29	13
Categories:				
- Physical abuse	9	7	6	1
- Sexual abuse	3	-	1	1
- Newborns 'at risk'	15	12	11	5
- Problems of care including neglect, emotional abuse and failure to thrive	9	15	7	6
Legal status:				
- Care Order	15	13		2
- Ward of Court	7	17	1	9
- Total (Percent of children)	22 (61%)	30 (77%)	25 (86%)	11 (85%)
Age on admission:				
- up to 1 month	10	10	9	6
- over 1 - 12 months	18	15	16	3
- over 1 - 5 years	8	11	4	4
- over 5 - 10 years	-	3	-	-
Admitted with:				
- mother only	12	18	10	10
- mother and father or partner	22	16	15	3
- siblings with parent(s)	2	5	4	-
Collaborative assessments of families with:				
- Clinical psychiatrist	1⎫	7⎫	6⎫	0⎫
- Child psychologist	0⎬ 15%	2⎬ 35%	5⎬ 60%	6⎬ 85%
- both [2]	4⎭	3⎭	4⎭	5⎭
Assessment by Adult Psychiatrist	9	4	1	-
Average length of stay	6 – 8 weeks			
Outcome for families:				
- discharged home	28 (78%)	26(67%)	20 (69%)	7 (54%)
- to foster care	8	13	9	6

1. Includes siblings
2, A psychiatrist from the Young Peoples Unit at Newcastle General Hospital also assessed two families in 1990

Table 18: Children with non-accidental fractures admitted to the Mother and Child Unit (FMH) and the Family Unit (NGH). 1978-1991 (up to 1 April)

Total number	26
Fractures (16 also had bruises)	13 (6 with limbs; 2 with subdural haematoma)
- Ribs	9
- Long bones	4
- Skull	
Age of injury	
- 3 months or less	16 (61.5%)
- Over 3-6 months	7
- Over 6 months	3
Legal status on admission	
- Care Order	16
- Supervision Order	4
- Ward of Court	4
- None	2 (the two parents responsible for the abuse were in prison)
Prosecution of parents	- 5 parents from 4 families - 3 fathers were jailed
Outcome ***On conclusion of residential assessment:***	
- Discharged home	17 ⎫ 69%
- To Mother and Baby Home	1 ⎬
- To foster care	8
After average of 16 months [1]	
- Still at home	15 ⎫ 58%
- To foster care [2]	2 ⎬

1. Range 4-5 months
2. One neglected, one with further bruising

150

Table 19: Non-accidental fractures. 1978 – 1 April 1991
Some factors associated with a failure to rehabilitate the children home to their families

	Total	Child to foster care after assessment
Previous history of parent in care	8	6
Parent(s) attended a special school for learning difficulties	6	4
Father with petty criminal record	6	5
Parents not married	15	8
Parents married *	7	2

* The five married parents who were able to continue to look after their children, all separated or divorced later in life

Table 20: Newborn babies 'at risk' of harm and neglect. Mother and Child Unit, Fleming Hospital and Family Unit, Newcastle General Hospital. 1978-1993

	1978-1989 [1], [2]	1989-1993
Total number	115	61
Legal order before assessment - total number - in 1989 - 1991 (N=35) - after 1991 - 1993 (N=26)	72 (63%)	33 (54%) 30 (86%) 3 (11.5%)
Average length of stay	6 weeks	6-8 weeks
On conclusion of assessment - discharged home - to foster care **After 12-18 months at home** - further number into foster care - total in foster care - total still at home	93 (80%) 22 (19%) 19 (16.5%) 41 (35.5%) 74 (64.5%)	43 (70%) 18 (30%)
First born baby – total number **On conclusion of assessment:** -discharged home - to foster care *After 12-18 months at home:* - further number into foster care - total number in foster care - total number still at home	58 (50%) 44 (76%) 14 (24%) 6 (14%) 20 (34%) 38 (66%)	22 (36%)
At least one previous child in care - total number *After home for 12-18 months:* - total in foster care - still at home	53 (46%) 21 (40%) 32 (60%)	35 (57%)

.   There is an overlap of 12 cases between these two periods, leaving a total of 164 between1978 and 1993
.   In 1978-1989, there was insufficient information in four cases for a classification of relevant antecedent factors

152

Table 21: 72 newborn babies 'at risk' at the Mother and Child Unit (Fleming Hospital). 1978 to mid-1987
Outcome related to some family 'risk factors'

	Number of newborns	In mid 1987	
		Still at home	In foster care
Severe learning difficulties* **- both parents** **- one parent**	14} 30 (42%) 16	4 12	10 (71%) 4 (25%)
Abuse or neglect of previous child	17	10	7 (41%)
Inability to care for previous children	16	8	8 (50%)
Mother aged 17 years or less	9	6	3 (33%)
Total	**72**	**40 (56%)**	**32 (44%)**

* Attended a special school

Table 22: Additional information about 61 newborns 'at risk'. 1989-1993

Reasons for residential assessment	
- Concerns about neglect or safe care in previous children	21
- Non-accidental injuries to previous children	18
- Mothers with first-born	
- concerns about mother's abilities	16
- father's past violent history	6 (27%)
Source of referral	
- maternity departments	44
- foster homes	8
- foster home with mother	3
- baby living with relatives	4
- mother and baby hostel	1
- mother and baby with friends	1
Legal orders before admissions	
1989 to 1991 (N=35):	
- Ward of Court	25 (71%)
- Interim Care Order	5
- No Legal Order	5 (14%)
1992 to 1993 (N-26):	
- Ward of Court	NONE
- Interim Care Order	3
- No Legal Order	23 (88%)
Number of previous children in care	
One child	14 ⎫
Two children	11 ⎬ 57%
More than two children	10 ⎭

Age of parents (years)	Mother	Father also resident
Up to 16	6 (10%)	
16-20	11	-
21-39	33	9
Over 30	11	27

Admission with parent(s)	
Mother only (father not involved)	18 (29.5%)
Mother only (father visiting)	7
Both parents	36 (59%)
Reasons for reception into care after admission (N=18)	
- Case conference recommendation – safe and effective care not possible	7
- Parents left, unable to complete assessment	5 ⎫
- Assessment discontinued due to disruptive behaviour of parents	5 ⎬ 55.5%*
- Baby accompanied by mother also on Care Order	1

* This represents a breakdown in the assessment in 16% of admissions

154

Table 23: History of sexual abuse in the childhood of mothers in a random
sample of records of families with issues of child protection.
1988-1991 (up to 1 April)

	Number of mothers	Sexual abuse in childhood
1988	34	3 (9%)
1989	34	5 (15%)
1990	25	12 (48%)
1991 (1 January to 1 April)	13	4 (31%)
Total	106	24 (23%)

155

Table 24: The honorary medical and surgical staff at the Babies Hospital.
1925 to 1945

		Later appointments in Newcastle
1925	Mr F.C. Pybus Dr G. Muir	Emeritus Professor of Surgery -
1927	Mr W.E.M. Wardill Dr S. Whateley Davidson	Consultant Surgeon Consultant Radiologist
1932	Dr A. G. Ogilvie Dr Elsie B. Wright	Consultant Physician Consultant Paediatrician
1934	Mr J.M. Saint	Senior Registrar in Surgery
1936	Dr G. Brewis	Consultant Paediatrician
1937	Dr Philip Ayre	Consultant Anaesthetist
1938	Dr F.J.W. Miller	Consultant Paediatrician Reader in Social Paediatrics
1940	Dr George Davison Mr Wm. Cowell	Consultant Paediatrician -

Dr A.F. Bernard Shaw, the pathologist who started post-mortems at the Babies Hospital in 1930, is not recorded as a member of the honorary staff. He later became Professor of Pathology at the Royal Victoria Infirmary.

Table 25: Problem families. List of 'deficiencies' recorded in the 1000 Family Study, Newcastle upon Tyne [14]

Mental deficiency (father or mother)

Mental illness (father or mother)

Serious physical illness (father or mother)

Prolonged or recurrent unemployment of wage-earner

No proper allowance to mother

Chronic family debt

Lack of minimal necessities in furniture and bedding

Gross lack of personal cleanliness

Domestic filth and disorder

Willful damage to property

Inadequate and irregular meals

Seriously defective clothing in children

Unnecessary crowding at night

Failure to call doctor for major illness

Failure to cooperate sensibly with health visitor, etc.

Leaving young children in charge of an inexperienced or unsatisfactory person

Truancy

Juvenile delinquency

Known and suspected cruelty or neglect

Parental crime

Excessive drinking (father or mother)

Excessive gambling (father or mother)

Excessive quarrelling (father or mother)

Sexual irresponsibility (father or mother)

Table 26: Families admitted to the Family Unit, Newcastle General Hospital, for
an assessment of the quality and safety of care.
1 April 1992 – 31 March 1994

Total number of families [1]	68
Admission of family with:	
- **one child**	58
- two children	8
- three children	2
Total number of children	80
- including siblings without injuries	4
Admission	
- with mother only	33
- with mother and current partner	35
Age of the children (including siblings)	
- up to 1 month	18 } 58%
- 1-6 months	28
- 6-12 months	14
- 1-2 years	10
- 2-3 years	5 } 13%
- 3-5 years	5
Families with previous children	
Total number	26 (38%) [2]

1. There is no information for one family
2. All the children are in the care of the local authority or other family members

Table 27: Age of the children at the time of the survey in July 1995.
The Family Unit, Newcastle General Hospital.
1 April 1992 – 31 March 1994

Under 2 years	7
2-3 years	13
3-4 years	27 } 69%
4-5 years	28
5-6 years	5

158

Table 28: Outcome in 80 children from 68 families admitted to the Family Unit at Newcastle General Hospital for an assessment of the quality and safety of the care of their children. 1 April 1992 – 31 March 1994

Initial outcome after assessment	
- home to care of parents	50 (62.5%)
- to another longer- care establishment with the parents for further assessment	3 [1]
- to grandparents	1
- to foster care	26 [2]
Outcome in July – August 1996 **2-4 years after residential assessment**	
- still at home	37 (46%)
- in care of local authority	16
- cot death	1
Legal orders on child still at home in 1996	
- none	32 (86%)
- full Care Order	4
- interim Care Order	1
Placement of children in care in 1996	
- with foster parent or families with a view to adoption	12
- adopted	9
- with family members	4 [3]
- returned home	1
Further assessment with a view to rehabilitation of children in foster care	10 [4]
Families with further children by 1996 after the end of the initial residential assessment	
- in families with children still at home	14 (38%) out of 37
- in families with children in foster care or adopted	7 (33%) out of 21

1. All three families failed to complete the assessment and the children went into foster care
2. The 26 children to foster care came from 46 families
3. One child with special needs lives with grandparents and the parents stay from time to time
4. One child who went home after the residential assessment, had a further injury (the severity is unknown)

159

Table 29: Responsibility and outcome in non-accidental injuries. The Family Unit, Newcastle General Hospital. 1 April 1992 – 31 March 1994

Total number	21[1]				
Number of uninjured siblings	4				
Responsibility for injuries:					
- unexplained	8				
- mother	7				
- father	6				
		At end of residential assessment		By 1996	
Injuries	Total	Discharged home	Foster care	Still at home	Foster care
Bruising only	6	4	2	4	2
Single fracture	2	2	-	1	1[2]
Multiple fractures	7	5	2	6 [3]	1
Single fracture and other injuries	6	3	3	2	(adopted) 4 [4]
Total	21	14 (**67%**)	7	13 (**62%**)	8
By 1996, placement of the children discharged home after a residential assessment:					
- with single mother				6	
- with both parents				3	
- with one parent after family split up				3	
- to foster care at request of their parents				2	

1. The majority were under the age of 1 year, with most under 6 months
2. Adopted later at mother's request
3. One child was eventually returned home after a further community assessment of the family
4. One child who went home after the residential assessment, had a further injury (the severity is not known)

160

Table 30: Newborn babies at risk admitted for a family assessment of the quality and safety of care by their family.The Family Unit, Newcastle General Hospital. 1 April 1992 – 31 March 1994

Total number	33
First child of the family - admitted with mother only - admitted with current partner - current partner who had previously injured or neglected his own child by another partner	5 3 3
Siblings - not cared for by their parents	22 **(67%)**

Outcome
After residential assessment
   -   discharged home
   -   to foster care
	
	25 **(76%)**
	8

By 1996 - still at home - in foster care - cot death	 15 **(45%)** 17* **(52%)** 1

*One child went into foster care following a further period of assessment based in the community after residence at the Family Unit

Table 31: Dysfunctional families admitted for assessment of quality and safety of care by their parents at the Family Unit.1 April 1992 – 31 March 1994

Total number	22
Number of families Admission with: - mother only - both parents	17 12 **(45.5%)** 5
Siblings (N=16) - not cared for by their family - help from grandparents	 3 1

Outcome
At the conclusion of the residential assessment:
  - home to parents
  - to foster care / adoptive parents
  - to other family members
	
	10 **(45%)**
	9*
	3

By 1996 - still at home - in foster care	 6 **(27%)** 1

* Further attempts at rehabilitation failed in two children

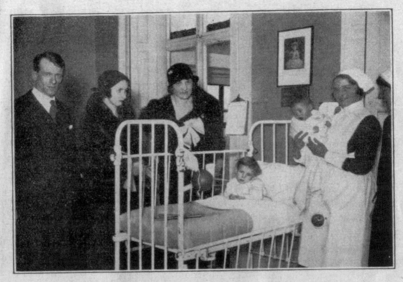

3

Reproduced by the courtesy of the Proprietors of the " North Mail" and " Chronicle."
Taken at the Annual Meeting on April 21st, 1932.

THE BABIES' HOSPITAL AND MOTHERCRAFT CENTRE.

SEVENTH ANNUAL REPORT,
April 1st, 1931, to March 31st, 1932.

In presenting the Seventh Annual Report of the Babies' Hospital the Committee desire to express their appreciation of all the help, monetary or otherwise, given them during the year. They also wish to thank all those who have served the Hospital in an Honorary capacity and especially the Honorary Medical Staff who have given much of their valuable time to the furtherance of the work.

The Committee is glad to report that in response to their invitation, Dr. Elsie Wright and Dr. Alan Ogilvie, have agreed to join the Honorary Staff.

The resignations of Mrs. Roy Williamson and Miss D. Richardson, from the Committee, owing to their removal from the town, are very much regretted. Their valuable help and wise counsel will be very much missed.

In order to be able to fill vacancies on the Committee which occur unexpectedly during the year, it has been decided to alter Rule 4 of the Constitution and add : " With power to co-opt." It has also been decided to increase the number of ordinary members to twelve.

Interesting visitors during the year have been Professor Ruston McIntosh, of New York, Dr. Brown of New Zealand and Professor Turverud of Oslo. On Christmas Day we also had a visit from the Lord Mayor and Lady Mayoress (Alderman and Mrs. Nixon) and Civic Party, which was very much appreciated.

As foreshadowed in the last report, increased accommodation has been secured, although it has not yet been possible to provide a modern building. By procuring the house next door to the Hospital it is now possible to admit 8 mothers with their infants. The importance of this addition cannot be over-estimated, and it is interesting to note that during the past two years, 47 infants have been admitted with their mothers for operation, all of whom have done well. Three wards for private patients have been opened where infants of those who are able to pay fees can be accommodated. They are received either alone or accompanied by their mother or Nanny. The fees charged are according to the circumstances of the patients.

An office has also been provided and a research laboratory and other minor improvements have been made which add considerably to the comfort and efficiency of the Hospital.

The post-graduate lectures given by Dr. Spence arranged by the Post Graduate Committee of the University of Durham College of Medicine have been held and have been well attended by 38 medical men in general practice from various parts of Yorkshire, Durham and Northumberland. Use has also been made of the opportunity offered to students and graduates to attend the Hospital rounds.

IN-PATIENTS. Particulars of the various and interesting cases admitted will be found in the medical report. The hospital serves the whole northern area as may be seen by the acompanying table which shows the sources from which the cases were derived. There were 21 infants and 1 mother in hospital on January 1st, 1931, and 222 have been admitted during the year, 28 of these were accompanied by their mothers. Mothers who were unable to leave their other children at night attended daily for feeding.

Newcastle	...	...	...	...	131
Northumberland	...	...	...	...	21
Durham County	...	...	...	...	29
Gateshead	...	...	...	...	9
Blyth	...	...	...	...	6
Bedlington	...	...	...	...	12
Newburn	...	...	...	...	4
North Shields	...	...	...	...	2
South Shields	...	...	...	...	2
Sunderland	...	...	...	...	1
Billingham	...	...	...	...	1
Stockton	...	...	...	...	2
West Hartlepool	...	...	...	...	1
Carlisle	...	...	...	...	1

As stated in former reports the Hospital has the approval of the Ministry of Health and works in sympathetic relations with the Health Departments of the City Council and the Councils of Northumberland, Durham, Blyth, Longbenton, Gosforth, Bedlington and Newburn, all cases admitted from their areas being reported to them. In the development of the Hospital the desire of the Committee is to work in the closest co-operation with existing Health services and other institutions in the district.

OUT-PATIENT DEPARTMENT. This Department is in constant use and the days on which patients may be seen has been increased to four. There have been 755 attendances during the year.

THE NURSING STAFF. The Matron, Miss Cummings, and her staff have carried on efficiently during the year, the Committee thanks them all for their interest and devotion to the Babies. Three Sisters who have been with us for periods varying from 2 to 3 years have now obtained posts at Great Ormond Street Hospital for Children, Vincent Square Babies' Hospital, London, and the Municipal Hospital for Babies at Birmingham ; the Committee wish them every success in their new posts. Nine probationers have completed their training during the year and have gained their certificates.

SEWING MEETINGS were again held at Miss D. Richardson's house, and she and her friends made the necessary garments and also did a quantity of mending. Another party is being formed by Mrs. Currie. Most valuable help has also been given by the Ryton Women's Institute, of which Mrs. Simpson is the President. The Committee is also grateful for the useful parcels of clothing received from the Northumberland Needlework Guild.

FINANCIAL REPORT. Attention is drawn to the Balance Sheet and Statement of Accounts. The overdraft unfortunately shows an increase, but when the extra provision made for the comfort of the patients and the staff is taken into consideration, the Committee feel that the expenditure is justified. Your attention is particularly drawn to the fact that the ordinary expenditure is less than the ordinary income, the cost per occupied bed, being approximately £2 : 3 : 4 per week.

Special efforts organised by the Committee include a Summer Market held by kind permission of Messrs. Fenwick, Ltd., in their Exhibition Hall, and a sale of " left-off " clothing.

A wireless appeal was also broadcast by the Chairman on March 20th.

The series of lectures which had unfortunately to be cancelled owing to lack of support, were not the heavy financial loss which was at first feared owing to the great generosity of the many friends of the Hospital who returned their re-funded ticket money.

A special Committee was formed to organise a Dance in the Old Assembly Rooms, with Mrs. T. Leathart as Chairman. The efficiency of Mrs. Wilson Brims and Miss Olive Willan as Honorary Secretaries largely contributed to its success.

As with all charities, the great need is for money, but should any sympathiser prefer to make gifts the immediate need of the Hospital is an X-Ray plant, at the cost of £200. Examinations of this type are largely used in all up-to-date Hospitals and at present patients have to be sent to other places to be photographed.

The success, if any, which attends this Hospital is the result of team work, the harmonious relations between the Hon. Physicians, Nursing Staff and Committee, being a most important factor for the welfare of the infants. The pace set by the Medical Staff is swift, without your aid we cannot keep pace with the ideal set by them.

URSULA RIDLEY (*Chairman*).

GRETA ROWELL (*Hon. Secretary*).

MEDICAL REPORT.

During the year ending 31st December, 1931, 222 infants were admitted as in-patients to the Hospital. At the beginning of the year there were 21 remaining in the wards. These make a total number of 243 infants treated as in-patients during the year.

The ages of the infants admitted were as follows :—

Under three months	65 cases
From four to six months	43 ,,
From seven to twelve months	53 ,,
Over twelve months	61 ,,

It is now seven years since the Hospital was opened. In each year the volume of the work has grown. An increasing demand is being made upon the Hospital for the admission of infants suffering from diseases of a severe and acute type. It is only those who are intimately associated with the work who can appreciate what is involved in the treatment, nursing and feeding of so many sick infants. Our experience is similar to that recorded from other infants' Hospitals, and shows that special arrangements are necessary in the care of the type of case with which we deal, and a method of staffing and nursing has to be developed— which throws a greater responsibility on Hospitals of this type than on Hospitals dealing with adults or older children. It is for this reason that the Committee has provided more accommodation for mothers who may be admitted with their infants and kept in Hospital when the establishment or continuation of breast feeding demands. The Honorary Medical Staff appreciates the keen insight and interest of the lay members of the Committee and of the Nursing Staff in dealing with these problems.

An analysis of the various diseases for the treatment of which the infants were admitted reveals that the commonest were as follows :—

Non-tuberculous lung diseases	38 cases
Tuberculosis	16 ,,
Sepsis and its effects	22 ,,
Gastro-intestinal diseases	18 ,,
Pyloric stenosis...	15 ,,
Pink Disease	14 ,,
Malnutrition	13 ,,
Rickets	11 ,,
Anæmia	9 ,,

The results reached in the cases discharged during the year were as follows :—

Recovered	151 cases
I.S.Q. and taken home or transferred ...	20 ,,
Died	48 ,,

An analysis of the fatal cases shows that 16 were admitted in a hopeless state of illness and died shortly afterwards. The causes of death were as follows :—

Broncho-pneumonia	12 cases
Tuberculosis	6 ,,
Gastro-enteritis	9 ,,
Convulsions	3 ,,

Pink Disease	...	...	...	...	4	cases
Sepsis with its effects	...	...	...	...	6	,,
Empyema	...	...	...	...	1	,,
Nephritis	...	...	...	...	1	,,
Hirschprungs Disease	...	...	...	...	1	,,
Congenital heart disease		...	...	...	1	,,
Uræmia	...	...	...	...	1	,,
Prematurity	...	...	...	...	1	,,
Bronchiectasis	...	...	...	...	1	,,
Pneumothorax		...	...	...	1	,,

The surgical work of the Hospital consists mainly of operations on special cases, especially infants with congenital abnormalities or suffering from Pyloric Stenosis. In this department special studies have been devoted to the problem of anæsthesia for these operations. We are glad to be able to record that these have given important results and have advanced considerably our knowledge of the use and control of anæsthesia in young infants.

A special clinic for the care and treatment of infants with hare lip and cleft palate is now being established. We expect that to yield good results, and the concentration of the work in it will give special opportunity for the study of the problems involved.

A feature of one of the problems of disease in infancy is revealed by the steady decline of infective gastro-enteritis in recent years, and a relative increase in diseases of the lungs, especially infective broncho-pneumonia. It is significant that whereas pneumonia is a frequent cause of death in ill nourished or improperly fed children it is rarely fatal amongst those who are well nourished and properly cared for. This reveals the great importance of an adequate and balanced diet in maintaining resistance to disease. On this point the experience of the medical staff is that the majority of the children, both from the towns and country districts, are not undernourished, but are improperly fed, due mainly to the excessive amount of cereal and bread which is provided in their diets. It is a danger that the people of this country eat too much wheat food to the exclusion of root vegetables.

With infants coming to the Hospital from many different towns and districts it has been possible to assess the great variation in the mother-craft of the women, that is in their capacity to care for and look after their infants. It is evident that the mother-craft of the urban mother is usually much below that of the mother from the outlying districts. It is particularly noticeable that the women from the Northumbrian villages, wives of miners and workers, inherit and maintain that capacity in high degree. They are well endowed with shrewd common sense and sagacity which makes good mothers of them.

As in previous years Post Graduate courses of instruction have been given in the Hospital by the Medical Staff. These have been attended by a larger number of doctors and students than ever before.

The Honorary Medical Staff has received valuable assistance from its Medical Officers Dr. Dorothy Holmes and Dr. J. R. Hindmarsh, and also from the clinical assistants who have been helping in the work.

The members of the Staff are anxious to acknowledge their gratitude to the Honorary Secretary and Members of the Committee, not only for their enthusiasm and help, but also for the efforts they make to keep in touch with new developments in the administration and management of hospitals of this type in this and other countries.

The Staff realises how much ultimately depends upon the skill and devotion of the Nursing Staff. It receives the most loyal co-operation from the Matron, the Sisters and the Nurses, and wishes to express its thanks to them. It is gratifying that the work of the Nursing Staff is widely recognised by a demand that is made for their services afterwards, and it is a matter for congratulation both for the Hospital and Sisters concerned that three of them have recently been chosen to fill appointments in three of the chief Children's Hospitals in England.

We are glad to record our thanks for the help and co-operation which we receive from our colleagues on the Medical Staffs of the local Public Health services, of other Hospitals in Newcastle and of the Newcastle Dispensary. By close contact with these every effort is made to co-ordinate our work and prevent overlapping. We have to acknowledge the help and advice of Dr. A. F. B. Shaw and of Professor Cornelia de Langa, of Amsterdam, in work undertaken in the pathological investigation of special cases.

This part of the report gives an opportunity for the Medical Staff to point out that there is a great need for help from individual donors who will give their money for the special purpose of endowing whole time workers to undertake special lines of research. The Hospital is equipped for this and affords special opportunities for it. There are two particular problems on which we have been able to throw some light—Pink Disease and tuberculous infection in early infancy. What is now required is that both of these should receive more intensive study by research workers, specially endowed to devote themselves to the work. It is hoped that some may realise the true economy of devoting money to these purposes, and the value of the results likely to accrue.

J. C. SPENCE, M.D., F.R.C.P.

Appendix 3

The finances of the Babies Hospital.1926-1945 Based on the accounts in the Annual Reports of the Hospital

	Total receipts (to nearest £)	Receipts as a % of the total				Donations and subscriptions [1]							Overdraft + = surplus - = deficit
		Ministry of Health	Newcastle City Council	Newcastle and northern districts	Mothers' fees	Total	% of total receipts	Total number of donations and subscriptions	Average individual amounts under £50	Donations and subscriptions of £50 or over			
										Number	Total	% of total	
1926-7	£4064	33%	3%		9.5%	£1190	29%	316	£2, 17s	4	£300	25%	+2%
1928-30	£6946	34%		14%	3.8%	£1243	18%	489	£2, 7s	2	£110	9%	-5.5%
1931-39	£29,086	-	-	43%	7.4% [2]	£7499	26%	1512	£3, 13s	29	£2980	40%	-11.4%
1940-44	£23,785 [3]	-	-	57%	4.3%	£7208 [4]	30%	775	£7, 12s	17	£1463	20%	-9.3%
Total	£63,881	-		42%	6%	£17,140	27%	3092	£4	52 [5]	£4853	28%	
1945	£7553	-		38%	-	£4202	56%	127	£4, 9s	6	£3660 [6]	87%	+67.4% [7]

1. Includes individuals, firms, schools, welfare centres and other charitable donation
2. The doubling of receipts from mothers' fees was associated with the opening of three private wards in 1932. Payment was 'according to circumstances'. Doctors' fees are not recorded

1. Includes a grant of £69 in 1944 from the Ministry of Health towards nurses' pay. Also, donations from the Admiralty towards the treatment of a patient - £58, 3s, 6p in 1941 and £59, 16s in 1942 and 1943
2. In order to repay an increasing overdraft, which reached £1275, 9s, 7p on the general account in 1940, Lady Ridley organised a special appeal: £561, 18s in 1940 and £581, 2s in 1941. As a result, the overdraft was reduced to £22, 3s, 6p in 1942. By 1944, it was again up to £123, 5s, 10p and was finally cleared in 1945
3. The number of donations and subscriptions of £50 and over represent only 1.7% of all donors providing about one-third of all donations
4. This includes a single legacy of £3000
5. This large surplus was due to the legacy of £3000, income tax recovered, bank interest allowed and the Bundle for Britain Fund from America

An estimate of the expenditure on each patient, based on the record of the annual expenditures [1] and the total number of inpatients each year, including new cases and those still in hospital from previous years.

	Total number of inpatients	Estimate of expenditure per inpatient [4]
1926-27	242	£16, 16s
1928-30	564	£12, 6s
1931-37 [2]	2262	£9, 10s
1940-43 [3]	1022	£18, 2s
1945	58	£34, 12s

1. The records indicate that the total expenditure each year was equal to the annual receipts as the accounts were always in balance

2 and 3. Information about the number of inpatients in 1938, 1939 and 1944 is limited to new admissions and does not include patients still resident from previous years. It has therefore been omitted for these years.

4. The cost of an occupied bed as distinct from the total cost of an inpatient admission rose from £2 6s 3p per week in 1931 to £4 6s in 1942

Notes:

- Earnings and living costs can provide a context in which the expenditures at the Babies Hospital may be evaluated.

- During the 1920s and 1930s up to 1938, the average earnings of employees in full-time employment in the main industries (excluding director' fees) were about 60 shillings a week with a range of 32 to 40s.[135] During the Second World War from 1940-1945, the average nominal weekly earnings were about 80 shillings, with little annual variation.[136]

- There were large differentials between the common forms of employment, as already indicated in the footnotes of Table A. In 1930, workers in agriculture and forestry earned an average of 30s per week, distribution trades 48s, mining and quarrying 54s, manufacturing 56s, building and contracting 60s, national government civil service 70s and insurance, banking and finance 101s.

- During the 1920s, it was estimated that 37s, 6p per week was necessary to achieve "a standard of bare physical efficiency" for a family of five. It was 53s in the 1930s "to secure the necessities of a healthy life" of such a family.[137]

- Many women in low income families had to seek employment to supplement their income. They were usually paid a great deal less than the men.

170

Appendix 4

James Spence's account of a 'typical' paediatric ward in c. 1944 -1946.
Transcript from "The Care of Children in Hospitals."
The Charles West Lecture. 1946.[27]

"It is easy to slip into satire to describe a children's ward, but the following is not far off the mark to many in our hospitals.

The room is vast. It contains twenty beds, spaced along walls tiled by Doulton or painted chocolate and yellow. The roof is remote – too remote for the cleaner's brush, and terrifyingly remote to the eyes of a child who lies many hours gazing at it.

Some of the beds are 3 feet from the ground, for the comfort of physicians and surgeons with ageing backs, but to the discomfort of the child who has not slept this far from the ground before. Many of these beds are protected by bars set close enough for protecting a child from lodging his head between and high enough to prevent him falling overboard. The beds stink just a little. Near the bed is a contraption, half-chair and half- locker, but it is beyond the reach of the child except by a contortion he cannot make so soon after his operation. He defeats this by concealing his personal treasures under his pillow until they are again put out of his reach. He solaces himself with comics or with paper and a scrubby pencil, which he cannot sharpen.

He dislikes the pallid immobile child in the next bed because he is too young for companionship or too ill for talk, but, as is the way of children, he makes the best of it and carries on a conversation with a boy of his own age 10 yards away over the heads of a whimpering baby and a plaintive a-year-old standing behind the bars of his cot with a loose napkin sunk to his ankles below. This child's plaint is not difficult to interpret. He draws the attention of a nurse busy with noughts and crosses on a temperature chart. She acts quickly and then goes to other duties in the kitchen, where she floats mashed potatoes on plates of liquid mince. The children await their dinner, but are distracted by strange events. A white-coated young man arrives and descends upon the silent occupant of a bed who, knowing that her penicillin hour is at hand, breaks her silence in a 4-hourly scream. The other distractions at other times – the daily or twice-weekly promenade of an older man in black with a retinue of followers; the occasional quick incursion of a younger man more sprucely clad, who pronounces his decision with a 'put on the list for next Tuesday'; the solemn visit of the matron, who passes from bed to bed with the same question on her lips at every bed; the arrival of an injured child at night; the piece of chocolate after dinner; the excitement of strange instruments which the doctors and nurses use but do not explain. Night comes on, but there is no bedtime story, no last moment of intimacy, no friendly cuddle before sleep. The nurse is too busy for that, busy with the noughts and crosses. This daily rhythm of anxiety, wonder, apprehension and sleep is better than it sounds, because it is made tolerable by the extraordinary resilience and gaiety of the children at every opportunity. Their cheerfulness keeps on breaking through. But it is a deceptive cheerfulness.

171

In the hospital there are other wards like this, with a kitchen, a side-room, a linen cupboard, and an entrance corridor beyond which parents shall not pass. They have no treatment room, no laboratory, no accommodation for parents, no interviewing room. Each ward is under a black-coated man of authority, who although devoted to his work, must delegate much of it to a white-coated resident. He has little time for companionship with his colleagues except in committee rooms. His ward is his domain. If he is a surgeon it is a surgical ward. If he is a physician it is a medical ward.

Not all hospitals are like this. Some are better, but many others are worse, mainly because most of the clinical work is in the hands of people untrained in paediatrics or insensitive to the fears of children. But I have drawn this picture in order to make concrete suggestions for its improvement."

Note:

J.C. goes on to make detailed practical proposals to resolve these issues. These include:

"In each unit, or conveniently near each unit, there should be a suite of special rooms in which, when necessary, a mother may live with, nurse, and care for her own child. She will do this under supervision of the trained staff. Five or more rooms of this sort will be required in a unit of fifty beds."

Appendix 5

The references of James Spence to earthworms, their significance and the naturalists who wrote about them.[120 and 121]

This refers to J.C.'s comments recorded in 'The Purpose and Practice of Medicine' (1960), pp. 177-178. [4]

Gilbert White FRS (1720-1793) was a "parson-naturalist", a pioneering English naturalist and ornithologist. He was born in his grandfather's vicarage in Selborne in Hampshire and remained a curate all his life. He is regarded by many as England's first ecologist. In a letter in 1777 he wrote:

"Earthworms, though in appearance a small and despicable link in the chain of nature, yet, if lost, would make a lamentable chasm…worms seem to be the great promoters of vegetation which would proceed but lamely without them…."

Darwin also had an interest in earthworms. He calculated that 53767 earthworms were recycling away per acre of arable land.

For J.C. earthworms appear to have provided him with a metaphor for 'industry' and 'utility'.

Appendix 6

Dr J. Robertson's account of the reaction of Dr Dermod MacCarthy to the film of 'A Two-year-old Goes to Hospital'. This consists of a transcript of the account in 'Separation of the Very Young' (1989) pp. 53-54. 94 [113]

In 1953, I met Dr Dermod MacCarthy, consultant paediatrican at Amersham Hospital. At the premiere of A Two-year-old Goes to Hospital at the Royal Society of Medicine in November 1952. He has been one of the many who were angered by the film, a humane paediatrician who felt that he and the profession were slandered.

Driving back to Amersham with his ward sister, Ivy Morris, he spoke crossly about 'Robertson', who had said such things about children in hospital. Sister Morris pulled him up with the words, 'But what Mr Robertson says is true'.

Next day Dr MacCarthy found, as he himself admitted, that he could no longer walk down his children's ward with his former complacency. He was suddenly aware of Lauras (the name of the child in the film 'A Two-year-old Goes to Hospital') among the younger patients. He wrote 'I was angry but after the film I really heard children crying for the first time'. Unlike some of his fellow paediatricians who remained angry and unchanged after the film presentation, Dr MacCarthy put his roused anxiety to good use. He had long been easy about visiting and occasionally had mothers stay, but now realised the full implications of the young child's need of the mother. He quickly opened the ward to unrestricted visiting and encouraged all mothers of under-fives to stay. He did not pick and choose between them on grounds that some were more suitable than others; family doctors in the community could tell the mother of any young child that they were sending to hospital that they could stay with him.

In the opinion of Dr MacCarthy and his like-minded colleagues, Sister Ivy Morris and Registrar Dr Mary Lindsay, the young patient needed his mother; no matter what the staff's view of her might be, their task was to get on with healing the illness and keep mother and child together.

Dr MacCarthy's relaxed ward was heart-warming to see. When brought fully into their children's care, most mothers were as competent and sensible on the ward as they were at home. The occasional one who was feckless or fearful got more nursing support, there was no question of excluding her. The anxiety about the mothers who fed sweets and cakes to their children had been dispelled; mothers whose affection and concern were not obstructed by restrictions had less need to bring sweets things. There was no increase in infections. Student nurses were a greater source of infection than were mothers to their children.

Notes:
Dr Mary Lindsay later went on to become a child psychiatrist.
Dr MacCarthy became a strong supporter of Dr Robertson. One of the influential films 'Going to Hospital with Mother' was made on his paediatric ward at Amersham Hospital and he became an adviser to the National Association for

the Welfare of Children in Hospital. (NAWCH). This Association was founded in 1961 following the publication of the Platt Report as 'Mother Care for Children in Hospital'; the name was changed to NAWCH in 1991.

He was also a strong supporter of child psychiatry. He convened the discussion group (attended by Dr Christine Cooper early in her career), which met regularly at Anna Freud's house in Hampstead and he was also a consultant paediatrican to the Institute of Child Psychology in London. [134]

In his report "The Emotional Well-being of Children Aged under 5 Years in Hospital."[122] Dr MacCarthy described five 'outworn' objections to the admission of mothers to hospital with their young children.

The mother's place is in the home. She cannot leave her other children.

The father will profit by the mother's absence to commit acts of infidelity.

In the presence of the mother, the child is more anxious and reacts badly to nurses and doctors, making examinations, diagnosis and treatment more difficult.

The mother's own anxiety upsets the child.

By dispensing with the mother, after a few days, a docile child.

He then describes ten good reasons for keeping mother and child together in hospital, with participation of the mother in nursing care:

Prevention of separation anxiety.

To diminish the probability of nervous upsets after hospital, by reducing stress.

To satisfy the mother's own need to stay with her sick child. (he quotes J.C.'s recommendation to this effect).

To hasten convalescence and early discharge of the patient.

To reduce cross infection. The mother disposes of all excreta and the child is handled by fewer nurses.

To teach the mother certain things (dressing, medicaments, diet etc.).

To observe the interaction of mother and child, many of whom are older rand more experienced in the simple care of babies and children than young nurses.

To observe the interaction of mother and child and see this in relation to the child's illness. The key to the problem is sometimes discovered in this way.

Handicapped children are specially dependent on the mother and may regress severely during a hospital experience without her. Children who cannot speak the language also need the mother.

To continue breast feeding.

Addendum. An obituary about a children's nurse, June Jolly SRN, RSCN, was published on the 12 April 2016 in the Telegraph newspaper. She had written an inspiring, innovative book entitled, 'The Other Side of Pediatrics. A Guide to the Everyday Care of Sick Children.' (1981). Figure 32. It contains a foreword by Dr MacCarthy. [139 a and b]

Appendix 7

Letter submitted to the inquiry on "The Welfare of Children in Hospital", chaired by Sir Harry Platt. 1957-1959.[117]

Transcript from James and Joyce Robertson. "Separation and the Very Young." Letter 11, pp.65-66.[113]

A year ago my daughter died in hospital at the age of 20 months. I was one of those mothers who was fortunate my baby did not go into hospital alone.

You probably know about this hospital but I will describe it from the mother's point of view. Small, wildly inconvenient for the nurses. Mothers and children in pleasant bed-sitters, unaccompanied children in cubicles or a smallish nursery. Meals for mothers – a cooked midday and evening meal, the makings of breakfast and tea, etc., and (a great boon) telephone which could be used at all times without troubling the staff. I shall never forget the kindness of the staff. I was filled with admiration for them all. Dr – who came in at 10 pm that night to see how Mary had settled: sister-in-charge, who was so kind and could inspire awkward mums with great respect, but who could allow informality and dignity.

It was through no fault of the hospital that things took the course they did. She thrived in the summer, and in the autumn she had a cough. The doctor sent us to the Babies Hospital for tests, which confirmed the suspicion of fibrocystic disease. The next stay for a fortnight was much more harrowing and worrying. We came home to carry out the treatment. A week later her chest became worse. She went back to hospital in an oxygen tent and died three days later – her heart gave out.

To have sent her into a ward alone might not have mattered much at two and a half months, but it would have been cruel at 19 months. She had been ill for 3 months and had my undivided attention all the time. To have been catapulted from that to loneliness would have been dreadful. As it was, although she fought the treatment all the time, and got frightened, I was with her and she had many happy hours right up to the last week.

Apart from the child, who is the prime consideration, the mother, too is better being with the child. You know what is going on and how things are. When things go badly mothers help each other. Without any conscious arrangement the mothers of dangerously ill and doomed children gravitate towards each other and we did get help from one another in different ways according to our natures.

We saw the work, tireless and unceasing, which went to help our children. I have seen doctors and nurses who were tired out after a heavy day return to deal with some problem. So I knew that if human endeavour could have saved my child, she would have lived, she would be living.

Because we knew the doctors so well, and saw them so often, we could feel like a family. When Mary died, Dr – was able to say things which were a real help and consolation. He couldn't have done so if we hadn't 'lived together'.

There were all kinds of mothers. What struck me was that the child wanted his mother, even if by my standards she was ghastly. One in particular was dreadful by any standard, but was there because her child had pined for her when there alone. He would rather have the mother who knocked him about than the kind conscientious and often dedicated nurses. There were other things that were not perfect. I won't bother to enumerate them, but I mention the fact in case you think that over enthusiasm has destroyed my power of judgement, but I would do anything to help popularise the idea of the Babies' Hospital.

Newcastle Babies Hospital.

REFERENCES

1. Lancet (1954). Obituaries, June 5, 12, 19, pp. 1190-94; 1247-1248; 1303.

2. British Medical Journal (1954). Obituary 5 June.

3. Ridley U. (1956). "The Babies Hospital Newcastle upon Tyne." Andrew Reid Company.

4. Charles J. (1960). Memoir in "The Purpose and Practice of Medicine." Selections from the writings of Sir James Spence, pp. 1-24. Oxford University Press.

    a. "Pink Disease", pp.71-79.

    b. "Investigation into the health and nutrition of certain of the children of Newcastle upon Tyne between the ages of one and 5 years", pp.142-158.

    c. "A clinical study of Xerophthalmia and night- blindness", pp. 49-50.

    d. "The purpose of the family: a Guide to the Care of Children", pp.174-203.

    e. "Family studies in preventive paediatrics", pp. 204-205.

5. Miller F.J.W. (1997). "Sir James Spence Kt MC MD LLD Durham Hon DSc FRCP, Professor of Child Health (1928-1954)." Journal of Medical Biography, 5 (1) pp.1-7.

6. "James Spence Medallists - Dr Frederick J.W. Miller." Archives of Disease in Childhood, 62, pp.766-767.

7a. Miller F.J.W. (1954), "James Spence and Social Paediatrics" in Gordon Dale and F.J.W. Miller (1984). "Newcastle School of Medicine, 1834-1984. Sesquicentennial Scrapbook", p 97. The Faculty of Medicine University of Newcastle upon Tyne.

7b. Miller F.J.W. (1990-1991). Unpublished memoir.

8. Ellis E. (c.1985). Unpublished memoir.

9. The Evening Chronicle (Newcastle-upon-Tyne) (1986). "First Steps in a Revolution. Baby Unit was the birthplace of many new ideas." May 23.

10. Court D. (1975). "Sir James Spence." Archives of Disease in Childhood, 50, pp. 85-90.

11. Annual Reports of the Babies Hospital and Mothercraft Centre, 33 West Parade, Newcastle-upon-Tyne. (1 April 1925 - 31 March 1937). The Babies Hospital, West Parade (1 April, 1937 - 31 December 1939) and the Babies Hospital, Blagdon Hall, Northumberland (1 January 1940 - 31 December 1945).

12. Bound Admission Records of the Babies Hospital. Leazes Terrace (1948 - 1976).

13. "The Mother and Child Unit, The Fleming Hospital. History, development and use." (1977-1985). Includes a memorandum by Dr Christine Cooper about the Wellburn Nursery at Ovingham, Northumberland.

14. Reports of the Family Unit at Newcastle General Hospital (1987-1991).

15. Dale G., Donald J. and Wagget J. (1987). "The Family Unity" and the "Nuffield Child and Psychology and Psychiatry Unit for Children and Young People" in "The Fleming Memorial Hospital for Sick Children. (1887-1987)", p 47.

(Note: 11, 12, 13, 14, 22 are held in the Tyne and Wear Archives and Museums. www.twomuseums.org.uk/tyne-and-wear-archives.html)

16. Spence J. (1920). "Some observations on sugar tolerance." Quarterly Journal of Medicine, 14, pp. 314-26.

17. Spence J. (1921.) "The use of laevulose as a test for hepatic inefficiency" (with P.C. Brett). Lancet, 201, pp. 1362-6.

18. Spence J.C., Walton W.S., Miller F.J.W. and Court S.D.M. (1954). "A Thousand Families in Newcastle upon Tyne." Oxford University Press.

19. "Infant Mortality Rate in Newcastle upon Tyne and England and Wales" in "A vision of Britain through Time", c. 1910-1970: GB Historical GIS/University of Portsmouth and Newcastle-upon-Tyne. http:/www.visionofbritain.orguk/unit/10108913/rate/INF_MORT

20. Kerr H. (1916). "Maternal and Child Welfare." Report of Medical Officer of Health. Newcastle upon Tyne. The Journal of the Royal Society for the Promotion of Health. 1 January.

21. Dwork D. (1987). "War is good for babies and other young children. A history of the infant and child welfare movement in England." (1898-1918). Chapter: "Infant Mortality and the future of the race", pp. 11-13. Tavistock Publications.

22. Annual Reports of the West End Day Nursery. 1919-1924.

23. Hill T. E. (1916). Medical Officer of Health, Durham Country. "Protection of Infant and Child Life" (in Darlington), p 61. Printed by North of England Newspaper Ltd. archive.org/stream/annotatedsubject00ameruoft _ djvu.txt

24. Report from the Babies' Nursery and Mothercraft Centre. West Parade.(1925).

25. Sir Truby King, (1923). "The Expectant Mother and Baby's First Months." pp. 32-40. Macmillan and Co. London.

26. Proud G. (2006). Chapter: "Surgery and Surgical Specialities" in "100 years of the RVI. 1906-2006", p 56. Editors Walton J. and Irving M. Newcastle upon Tyne NHS Trust.

27. Spence J. (1947). The Charles West Lecture. Royal College of Physicians. London. "The Care of Children in Hospital." British Medical Journal, 1, pp. 125-131.

28. Spence J.C. and Miller F.J.W. (1941). "Causes of Infant Mortality in Newcastle upon Tyne. 1939." Newcastle Health Committee.

29. Morley M.E. (1945). "Cleft Palate and Speech." Churchill Livingstone.

30. Morley M.E. (1957). "The Development and Disorders of Speech." Churchill Livingstone.

31a. "The Development of Speech Therapy in Newcastle" and "From Speech Therapy Clinic to Academic Sub-Department." (2009). University of Newcastle upon Tyne.

31b. "Brief History. School of Education Communication and Language Sciences" http;//www.ncl.ac.uk/ecls/about/subjectareas/speechlanguage/history.htm

32. Dally A. (1997). "The rise and fall of Pink Disease." Social History of Medicine, 10/02, pp. 291-305.

33. Spence J. (1933). "Clinical Tests of the Antirachitic Activity of Calciferol." Lancet, 225, p 1911.

34 a. Spence J. (1932). "Benign Tuberculous Infiltration of the Lung. ("Epituberculosis")." Lancet, 7, no. 37, February 1932, 1.

34 b. Miller F.J.W., Seal R.M.E., Taylor M.D. (1963). "Tuberculosis in Children." J.A. Churchill.

34 c. Miller F,J.W. (1982). "Tuberculosis in Children. Evolution, epidemiology, treatment, prevention." Medicine in the Tropics. Churchill Livingstone.

35. Brewis E.G., Davison G. and Miller F.J.W. (1940). "Investigation of the health and nutrition of certain of the children of Newcastle upon Tyne between the ages of 5 years (1938-39), City and County of Newcastle upon Tyne." Newcastle Health Department.

36. Lomax E.H.R. (1996). "Small and Special. The Development of Hospitals for Children in Victorian Britain." Medical History, Supplement No. 16, pp. 4 and 36. Wellcome Institute of the History of Medicine. London.

37. Hurrel G., Harbon G.P. (Reprinted 1984). "The History of Newcastle General Hospital. 1870-1966", p 16. Henderson and Co. Ltd.

38. Tacchi D. (1994). Chapter: "The Paediatric Contribution (1942-1990)" in "Childbirth in Newcastle upon Tyne (1760-1990)", p 116. Berwick Press.

39. Miller F.J.W., Court S.D.M., Walton W.S, and Knox E.G. (1960). "Growing up in Newcastle upon Tyne." Oxford University Press.

40. Miller F.J.W., Court S.D.M., Knox E.G. and Brandon S. (1974). "The School Years in Newcastle upon Tyne." Oxford University Press.

41. Kolvin I., Miller F.J.W., Scott D. Mcl., Gatzanis S.R.M. and Fleeting M. (1990). "Continuities of Deprivation? The Newcastle 1000 Family Study." Avebury.

42. Mark S Pearce, Nigel C Unwin, Louise Parker and Alan w Craft. (2009). "Cohort Profile: The Newcastle Thousand Family 1947 Cohort." International Journal of Epidemiology, 38, pp.932-937.

43. Pearce M.S. (2008-2015) Joint author in publications related to the 1000 Family Studies, Newcastle upon Tyne. Pubmed pearce ms

44. Pearce M.S., Mann K.D., Relton C.L., Francis R.M., Steele J.G., Craft A.W., Parker L. (2012). "How the Newcastle Thousand Families birth cohort study has contributed to the understanding of the impact of birth weight and early life socioeconomic position on disease in later life." Maturitas, May, 72(1), pp. 23-28.

45. Craft A.W. (2003). "Fetal programming or adult life style. Lessons from the 1000 Families Study." `Hong Kong Journal of Paediatrics, 8, pp.346-353.

46a. Paediatric and Lifecourse Epidemiology Research Group. Newcastle University. "1000 Families Study -50 Years Old in 1997."http://research.ncl.ac.uk/plerg/Research/1000F/1000ages50.htm

46b. Parker, L, Lamont D.W., Wright O.M., Cohen M.A., Alberti K.G.M., and Craft A.W. (1999). "Mothering skills and health in infancy. The Thousand Families Study revisited. *The Lancet*, 353, pp 1151-2

47. Spence J. (1938). "The Modern Decline of Breast-feeding." British Medical Journal, 2, p 729.

48 Spence J.C. (1940). "The Nation's Larder in Wartime." British Medical Journal, July 30, pp. 93-95.

49. "The famine of 1944 (Netherland). http:/en.wikipedia.org/wiki/Dutch_famine_of_1944

50, Angell-Anderson E., Tretli S., Bjerknes R., Forsen T., Sorensen T.I.A., Eriksson J.G., Rasanen L. and Grotmol T. (2004). "The association between nutritional conditions during World War II and childhood anthropometric variables in the Nordic countries." Annals of Human Biology. (May-June 2004), Vol. 31, No.3, pp. 342-355.

51. "Wartime rationing helped the British get healthier than they had ever been", in Medical News Today. A MediLexicon International Report last updated 21 June 2004.

52. Spence J. 1946. The Convocation Lecture of the National Children's Home in "The Purpose of the Family: a Guide to the Care of Children." Chapter in "The Purpose and Practice of Medicine." Oxford University Press. (1960), pp. 174-203.

53. Dr Christine Cooper (1918-1986). Munks Roll. Royal College of Physicians of London.

54. Court S.D.M. (1986). An address, "In Memory and Friendship" at a memorial service in honour of Dr Christine Cooper.

55. Houghton W. (1972). "Report of the Departmental Committee on Adoption of Children." Comnd 5107. HMSO.

56. Helfer R.E. and Kempe C.H. (1968). "The Battered Child." First Edition. The University of Chicago Press.

57 Lynch M.A. (1985). "Child abuse before Kempe: an historical literature review." Child Abuse and Neglect, Vol. 9, pp. 7-15.

58. Kempe C.H., Silverman F.N., Steele B.F., Droegemueller W. and Silver H.K, (1962). "The battered child syndrome." Journal of the American Medical Association, 181, pp.17- 24

59. Hobart C., Frankel J. (2005). Chapter: "The history of child abuse" in "Good Practice in Child Protection." 2nd Edition, pp. 1-16. Nelson Thornes Ltd.

60. Obituary. Dr Christine Cooper. (1986). The Lancet. September 20, pp. 699-670.

61. Cresy Channan. (1992). "Changing Families: Family Centres. Changing Welfare. Family Centres and the Welfare State", pp. 4-5 and 57-62. Harvester Wheatsheaf.

62. Cooper C.E. (1985). Chapter: "Good-enough, Borderline and Bad-enough Parenting." In "Good-enough Parenting – a framework for assessment." Edited by Adcock M. and White R. Published by British Agencies for Adoption.

63. Pullan C.R., Dellagramatikas H. and Steiner H. (1997). "Study of gastro-enteritis in children admitted into hospital in Newcastle upon Tyne. British Medical Journal, 1, pp. 619-621.

64. Klaus M.H., Kennell J.H. (1976). "Maternal – Infant Bonding." C.V. Mosley. Saint Louis.

65. Lynch M.A., Roberts, J. (1977). "Predicting child abuse: signs of bonding failure in the maternity hospital." British Medical Journal, 1, pp. 624-626.

66. Weaver L., Steiner H. (1984). "The Bowel Habit of Young Children." Archives of Disease in Childhood, Vol. 59, no. 7, pp. 649-652.

67. Neligan G., Prudham D., Steiner H. (1974). "The Formative Years. Birth, family and development in Newcastle upon Tyne." Published for the Nuffield Provincial Hospitals Trust by Oxford University Press.

68. Steiner H. (1975). Chapter: "Paediatrics in Hospital and Community in Newcastle upon Tyne." In "Bridging in Health. Reports of studies in health services for children." Published for the Nuffield Provincial Hospitals Trust by Oxford University Press.

69. Steiner H. (1986). Abstract: "Assessment and help for families with psycho-social problems in the parent and child unit of a children's hospital." Proceedings of the 58th Annual Meeting of the British Paediatric Association. York 15-18 April.

70. Steiner H. (1990). Abstract: "The prospects of rehabilitation of infants with non-accidental injuries." 62nd Annual Meeting of the British Paediatric Association. 3-6 April.

71a. Report on a family training centre in Newcastle. (1983). "Parenting – we're being allowed to keep him." Community Care, 21, pp. 15-17.

71b. Obituary, Mr Brian Roycroft. The Guardian 31 May 2002.

72. Fairburn A.C., Trendinnick A.W. (1980). "Babies removed from their parents at birth. 160 Statutory care orders." British Medical Journal, 5 April, pp. 987-991.

73. Freedman, M.D.A. (1980). "Removing Babies at Birth. A questionable practice." Family Law, April, pp. 131-134.

74. Cooper C.E. (1979). "Babies at risk." British Medical Journal, 29 September, p. 792.

75. Steiner H. (1990). Abstract: "The safeguard of newborn babies at risk of harm and neglect." 62nd Annual Meeting of the British Paediatric Association. 3-6 April.

76. Greenacre E. M. (1995). "Can we keep him?." Dissertation submitted for qualification during a course of the English National Board on Child and Adolescent Health (Course 603).

77. Shared Parenting Information Group (SPIG) UK. www.spig.clara.net

78. White R., Carr P., Lowe N. (1995). "The Children Act (1989) in Practice", pp. 6, 7, Section 1.20. Butterworths.

79. Mordue A. (1988). "An epidemiological study of suspected cases of child sexual abuse diagnosed in Cleveland" A report submitted for the MFCM Part II Examination. (Initially commissioned by the Regional Medical Officer, Dr Liam Donaldson.)

80. Wright C.M. (2005). Memorandum on "The Northumbria Women Police Doctors."

81. Report of the Inquiry into Child Abuse in Cleveland. 1987. HMSO.

182

82. Kolvin I., Steiner H., Bamford F., Taylor M., Wynne J., Jones D. and Zeitlin H. (1987). "Child Sexual Abuse: principles of good practice." British Journal of Hospital Medicine, Vol. 39, pp. 54-62.

83. Steiner H., Taylor M. (1988). "Description and Recording of physical signs of suspected child sexual abuse." British Journal of Hospital Medicine, Vol. 40, pp. 346-350.

84. San Lazaro C., Steel A.M. and Donaldson L.J. (1996). "Outcome of clinical investigations into allegations of sexual abuse." Archives of Disease in Childhood, 15,pp. 149-152.

85. Lazaro C. (2014). Personal communication.

86. Greenacre E. (Senior Sister at the Family Unit, Newcastle General Hospital), Fundudis T. (Consultant Clinical Psychologist) and Kaplan C. (Consultant Child Psychiatrist). (2014). Personal communications.

87. Greenacre E. et al (1996). Unpublished survey of outcome of children admitted to the Family Unit at Newcastle General Hospital Unit during 1992-1994.

88. Hobbs C.J., Helga G., Hanks I., Wynne J.M. (1999). "Child Abuse and Neglect. A Clinician's Handbook." Chapter: "Fatal Child Abuse", p. 440. Churchill Livingstone.

89. "Protecting Children. A guide for social workers undertaking a comprehensive assessment." (1988). H.M.S.O.

90. Dale F., Davies et al (1986). "Dangerous Families." Routledge.

91. Stones C. (1994). "Focus on Families, Family Centres in Action." Barnados Practical Social Work Series. Macmillan.

92. Turner S. (1982). "The Riverside Child Health Project." Evaluation Report. Department of Family and Community Medicine. University of Newcastle upon Tyne.

93. Downham M. (2014). Personal communication.

94. The Family Resource Team. (1997). First Annual Report. Newcastle upon Tyne Social Services Department.

95. "Fit for the Future" (1976). The Report of the Committee on Child Health Services. Volume I, pp.110-111 and 307-308, HMSO.

96. "Strengthening the care of children in the community. A Review of Community Child Health in 2001." Published by the Royal College of Paediatrics and Child Health.

97. Spence J. (1949). "Family Studies in Preventative Paediatrics." The Cutter Lecture on Preventive Medicine at the Harvard School of Public Health. In "The Purpose and Practice of Medicine", pp. 206-207 (1960). Oxford University Press.

98. Craft A. (2006). Chapter: "Children at the RVI." In "100 years of the RVI 1906-2006", p 102. Published by Newcastle upon Tyne NHS Trust.

99. Stephenson T. (2010). "NHS neglects parents of sick children." From the President of the Royal College of Paediatrics and Child Health. The Observer, 14 March.

100. Schapira K (2014). Personal communication.

101a. Gordon Dale and F.J.W. Miller (1984). "Newcastle School of Medicine. 1834-1984. Sesquicentennial Scrapbook." The Faculty of Medicine Newcastle University.

Walton J. "Some reflections of the class of '45", p. 88 Lowdon A.G.R. "New Medical Curriculum", p.110

101b. Walton J. (1993). "The Spice of Life", pp. 88-89. Royal Society of Medicine Services.

102. Scott J.E.S. (2006). Chapter: "The Associated Hospitals."In "100 Years of the RVI. 1906-2006", p 138. Published by Newcastle upon Tyne Hospitals NHS Trust.

103. Cooper C. (1978). "Seeing the Baby." Adoption and Fostering, 93, pp. 49-55.

104. Mary Bell. en.wikipedia.org.uk/wiki/Mary_Bell

105. Sereny, G. (1995). "The Case of Mary Bell. A portrait of a child who murdered", p 193. Pimlico.

106. Sereny, G. (1998). "Cries Unheard." The Story of Mary Bell. p 332. Macmillan.

107. John Bowlby. en.wikipedia.org.uk/wiki/John Bowlby.

108. Hobbs, C.J., Helga G., Hanks, I., Wynne, J.M. (1999). Chapter: "Emotional Maltreatment" in "Child Abuse and Neglect. A Clinician's Handbook", pp. 149-164. Second Edition. Churchill Livingstone.

109. Death of Maria Colwell. en.wikipedia.org/wiki/Death of Maria Colwell.

110. Hendrick H. (1997). Chapter: "Children and Social Policies" in "Children, Childhood and English Society, 1880-1990", pp. 36-62. Cambridge University Press.

111. The Curtis Report.(1946). In "History of Foster Care in England and Wales, 1946-1989." Grahamtaylor0.tripod.co

112. Nursing Times. (1952). "Visits to Children in Hospital." March 15.

113. James and Joyce Robertson. (1989). "Separation and the Very Young", pp.19, 23, 45, 53-54. Free Association Books. London.

114. Bowlby, J. (1951). "Maternal Care and Mental Health." WHO Monograph Series 2. HMSO.

115. Bowlby, J. (1997). "Attachment and Loss, Vol. 1, in "Attachment." Second Edition. Pimlico.

116. McCleod, S. (2009). "Attachment Theory." Retrieved from http://www.simplypsychology.org/attachment.html

117. The Platt Report. (1959). "The Welfare of Children in Hospital." DHSS.

118a. Hotherstall, D. (1984). "Sigmund Freud (1856-1939)" in "History of Psychology", pp. 215-228.Temple University Press. Philadelphia.

118b. Dr Carole Kaplan (2015). Personal communication.

119. Court D. and Jackson A. Editors. (1972). "Paediatrics in the Seventies. Developing the child health services", pp. 23, 45, 85-87. Published for the Nuffield Provincial Hospitals Trust by the Oxford University Press.

120. Gilbert White. Letter to the Honourable Daines Barrington. May 20,1777. In "The Natural History of Selborne." Edited by Anne Secord, letter 35, pp.172-3. Oxford University Press.

121. Charles Darwin. "The formation of vegetable mould through the action of worms." Section on "Renewed work on earthworms." http://en.wikipedia.org/wiki/Charles_Darwin

122. MacCarthy, D. (1982). "The emotional well-being of children under 5 years in hospital", pp. 3, 7-11. Third Edition, published first in 1979 by NAWCH. Originally requested by the Confederation of European Societies of Paediatricians of the European Economic Union and presented at a meeting of the confederation in 1973.

123. Joyce Robertson. Personal communication to Professor Sir Alan Craft in 2015.

124. The Observer, Sunday, 15 February 2015. "Giving a voice to dementia sufferers. How our campaign has built awareness." http://guardian.newspaperdirect.com/epaper/iphone/homepage.aspx#_arti cle156f8f1b-2957-465b-9b64-aea54af57816/waarticle156f8f1b-2957-465b-9b64-aea54af57816/156f8f1b-2957-465b-9b64-aea54af57816//true

125. Christopher Hobbs, Helga G. I. Hanks, Jane M. Wynne (1999). Chapter: "Sexual abuse: the scope of the problem", pp. 165-189 in "Child Abuse and Neglect. A Clinician's Handbook." 2nd Edition. Churchill Livingstone.

126. Broadhurst K., Harvin J., Shaw M., Abrouh B. (2014). "Capturing the scale and pattern of recurrent care proceedings: initial observations from a feasibility study." Family Law, August.

127. Rutter M. (1981). "Maternal Deprivation Reassessed." (2nd Edition). Harondsworth. Penguin Books.

128. Rutter M. (1985). "Resilience in the face of adversity: protective factors and resistance to psychiatric disorder." British Journal of Psychiatry, 147, pp. 591-611.

129. David M. Brodzinsky (1993). "Long-term Outcomes in Adoption" in The future of Children. ADOPTION. Vol. 3, N.1, Spring 1993.

130. Madge, N. (1983). "Families at Risk", p. 198. Heinemann Educational Books. London.

131. Lynch M., Steinberg D., Ounsted C. (1975). "Family Unit in a children's psychiatric hospital." British Medical Journal, 2, pp. 127-129.

132. Craft A.W. (2007). " Working together to protect children: who should be working with whom?" Archives of Disease in Childhood, 92 (7), pp. 571-573.

133. Seymour Donald Mayneord Court. Munks Roll, Royal College of Physicians of London. http://munksroll.rcplondon.ac.uk/Biography/Details/1030

134. Dermod De La Chevallerie MacDermid. (1911-1986). Munks Roll. Royal College of Physicians of London. Volume 8, p. 300.

135. Agatha L. Chapman and Rose Knight (1953), "Wages and Salaries in the United Kingdom (1920-1938)", pp. 27,30. Cambridge University Press.

136. The Annual RPI and Average Earnings for Britain, 1209 to Present. (New Series). http://www.measuringworth.com/datasets/ukearncpi/result2.php

137. Theo Barker and Michael Drake. (1982). "Population and Society in Britain 1850-1980", pp.144-145. New York University Press.

138. Dr John Scott Inkster. Obituary (2011). Association of Paediatric Anaesthetists of Great Britain and Ireland.
http://www.apagpi.org.uk/about-us/membership/obituaries/dr-john-scott-inkster
139[a.] June Jolly (1981) 'The Other Side of Pediatrics. A Guide to the Everyday Care of Sick Children.' University Park Press. Baltimore.
139[b.] Obituary. June Jolly. The Telegraph. 12 April 2016

INDEX

Court, D. C. M. – professor of child health 1, 23, 49, 52, 56, 88, 105, 106, 108, 109, 121, 123, 129-130
Cummings, Miss – matron Babies Hospital 24, 33

Darwin, C. – naturalist and geologist 121, 173
Donald Court – Chair of Community Child Health 130
Donaldson, Professor Sir Liam – Northern Region Medical Officer 81, 130
dyspepsia 25

education
    junior doctors 62
    medical students 16, 31, 32, 39, 47, 56, 62, 108, 109
    mothers 7, 16, 37, 105
    probationers / nurses 7, 16, 31, 32, 39, 62, 108
    postgraduate doctors 31, 32, 39, 47, 62, 108, 109
emotional needs of children
    Bowlby, J. – psychiatrist 115-117, 119, 123
    Court, D. C. M 123
    Cooper, C. 123
    McCarthy, D. – paediatrician 122, 123, 175
    Robertson, James – psychologist 113-115, 119-123
    Spence, James 14, 47, 104, 116-119, 121, 122, 171, 172

feeding difficulties 6, 8, 24, 25, 30, 37, 41, 105
finances of Babies Hospital 32-34, 128, 169, 170

good-enough parenting 53, 73, 110
Greenacre, E. – nursing sister 59, 84

Hey, E. – paediatrician 57
Hill, T. E. – medical officer 6

infant mortality rate 3, 19, 20, 29, 38, 40, 45
infections 10, 18-20, 38, 40, 42, 49, 105, 106, 108, 109
    tuberculosis 1, 27, 28, 40, 42, 49

Jackson, S. – social worker 60
Jolly, June – nurse 175
Joseph, Sir Keith – Secretary of State for Social Services
    cycle of deprivation 127

Kerr, H – Medical Officer of Health Newcastle upon Tyne 3-5
Kolvin I. – professor of child psychiatry 81, 123, 124

Lazaro, C – Senior Paediatric Registrar (later Consultant in
    Forensic paediatrics) 81
length of hospital stay 29, 37, 61, 73, 84

longstay inpatients 42, 117, 118
Lynch, M. – paediatrician 127

marasmus / malnutrition 8-12, 18, 19, 24, 28, 36, 40, 105
massage 10, 26
Medical Research Council 2, 26, 27, 40, 47, 107
milk
    human-certified sources 7, 12
    humanised 7, 12
    national milk scheme (World War II) 45
Miller, F. J. W. – reader in social paediatrics 1, 33, 38, 45, 46, 49, 109
    Infant mortality survey 20
    1000 families study 20, 38, 129
    tuberculosis 28, 106
Ministry of Health 11, 14, 32-35, 41, 45, 120, 128
miscellaneous medical conditions 17, 18, 38
Morley, M – speech therapist 23, 24
multidisciplinary arrangements 58-61, 65, 83, 84, 110, 121
Muir, G. – medical officer 7

National Society for the Prevention of Cruelty to Children 52-54, 60, 78-81, 112,
    127
nervous diseases 41
Newcastle City Council 4, 32-34, 104, 128
Newcastle General Hospital 35-37, 43, 52, 62, 73, 74, 76, 84, 110, 128
Newcastle upon Tyne, 1000 families studies 1, 3, 20, 38, 39, 54, 55, 106, 126
Nuffield Chair of Child Health 46, 47
Nuffield Psychology and Psychiatry Unit for Children
    and Young People 60, 67, 69, 73, 83, 84, 124
nutrition 19, 26, 44, 45, 48, 55, 105

pink disease (erythroedema) 17, 19, 24-26, 29, 41, 49, 107
Platt Report – Welfare of Children in Hospital 120, 123, 124
post-mortems 29
private patients 3, 11, 28, 31, 34, 103, 105
probationers 7, 32, 33
public bodies 32, 47
Pybus, F. C. – surgeon 13, 14

radiology 28
rickets 6, 8, 10-12, 17, 40
    treatment 14, 26, 27, 30
Ridley, U. – management committee 1, 14, 16, 29, 30, 33, 34, 41, 105
Rowell, G. – founder of West End Day Nursery 3, 5, 33
Roycroft, B – Director of Social Services, Newcastle upon Tyne 75, 76
Rutter, H L – General Practitioner and Medical Officer 5-7

Schapira, K. – psychiatrist 108
Shaw, A. F. B. – pathologist 2, 29
Steiner, H. – paediatrician 60, 83
Strang, L. – paediatric registrar. Later Professor of Paediatrics at
    University College Hospital, London 50
surgery 21-24, 41, 47, 49, 50, 57, 105, 109
    cleft palate and hare lip 21-24, 31, 50, 105
    newborn 50

Taylor, Margaret – paediatrician 81, 82
Taylor, Mary – paediatrician 43

visitors to the Babies Hospital 31, 49, 109

Walton, Lord John iv, 107, 109
Wardill, W. E. H. – surgeon 22-24, 40, 41, 48
Weaver, L. – paediatric registrar. Later Professor of Paediatrics,
    Glasgow University 58
Wellburn Residential Nursery 55
Whateley, Davidson – radiologist 28
White, G – naturalist 121, 173
World War II 17, 34, 35, 41-46, 103, 128
Wright, E. – paediatrician 23, 43, 52